CARDIOVASCULAR MULTIDETECTOR COMPUTED TOMOGRAPHY ANGIOGRAPHY

CARDIOVASCULAR MULTIDETECTOR COMPUTED TOMOGRAPHY ANGIOGRAPHY

Subha V. Raman MD
Division of Cardiovascular Medicine
Ohio State University
Columbus, Ohio
U.S.A.

Patricia V. Grodecki MD
Cardiology Associates, PSC
Edgewood, Kentucky
U.S.A.

Stephen C. Cook MD
Division of Cardiovascular Medicine
Ohio State University
Columbus, Ohio
U.S.A.

Mario J. Garcia MD
Mount Sinai Medical Center
New York, New York
U.S.A.

informa
healthcare

First published in the United Kingdom in 2007 by Informa Healthcare, 4 Park Square, Milton Park, Abingdon, Oxon OX14 4RN. Informa Healthcare is a trading division of Informa UK Ltd. Registered Office: 37/41 Mortimer Street, London W1T 3JH. Registered in England and Wales number 1072954.

Tel: +44 (0)20 7017 6000
Fax: +44 (0)20 7017 6699
Email: info.medicine@tandf.co.uk
Website: www.informahealthcare.com

A CIP record for this book is available from the British Library.
Data available on application

ISBN-10: 1-84184-645-7
ISBN-13: 978-1-84184-645-3

Distributed in North and South America by
Taylor & Francis
6000 Broken Sound Parkway, NW, (Suite 300)
Boca Raton, FL 33487, USA

Within Continental USA
Tel: 1 (800) 272 7737; Fax: 1 (800) 374 3401
Outside Continental USA
Tel: (561) 994 0555; Fax: (561) 361 6018
Email: orders@crcpress.com

Distributed in the rest of the world by
Thomson Publishing Services
Cheriton House
North Way
Andover, Hampshire SP10 5BE, UK
Tel: +44 (0)1264 332424
Email: tps.tandfsalesorder@thomson.com

Composition by Egerton + Techset
Printed and bound in India by Replika Press Pvt. Ltd.

Contents

Preface

Cardiovascular medicine has witnessed significant progress over the past century, incorporating the technical advances of each era to improve patient care. The introduction of the stethoscope, electrocardiography, roentgenography, angiography, invasive hemodynamics, ultrasonography, nuclear scintigraphy, and magnetic resonance have each, in turn, allowed progressively greater accuracy and precision in the diagnosis and treatment of cardiovascular disease. The advent of multidetector computed tomography using 64 detector rows and beyond provides the next leap forward in cardiovascular care, delivering on the promise of high-resolution visualization of cardiovascular structure and function noninvasively.

The goal of this book is to demonstrate the clinical context within which this technology is useful for individual patient assessment, while providing relevant technical information needed to perform cardiovascular multidetector computed tomography. Practicing clinicians know that patient care without technology is feasible, but medical technology applied without clinical acumen is, at best, irrelevant. Thus, in preparing this book we sought to demonstrate the application of cardiovascular multidetector computed tomography from the perspective of the care of the patient. We hope that this book is useful for cardiologists and radiologists alike, as well as primary care physicians, house officers, medical students, and other health care professionals who have the opportunity to use this exciting new technology to improve diagnosis and treatment for their patients with cardiovascular disease.

The authors wish to acknowledge the following individuals for their contributions: Ogei Yar, MD; Sanjay Patil, MD; and Silpa Kilaru, BS. We gratefully acknowledge the editorial feedback from Sandra S. Halliburton, PhD, to the chapter on artifacts. A special thanks is extended to Tam Tran, BS, whose sincere efforts throughout this project were invaluable.

Subha V. Raman
Patricia V. Grodecki
Stephen C. Cook
Mario J. Garcia

Chapter 1 Introduction

Computed tomography (CT) is a well-established technology for imaging based on the principle that an x-ray source and an array of detectors rotating around a target (patient) generate a set of attenuation information that, through filtered backprojection reconstruction algorithms, provides the mathematical basis to generate a cross-sectional image. Spiral CT involves moving the rotating x-ray source and the detector array as the table advances to cover a volume of tissue in the z (patient) direction (**Fig. 1.1**), thus creating a spiral trajectory. Adding multiple detectors along the z-axis allows generation of multiple slices of axial image information during a single rotation of the gantry (source–detector hardware). Greater z-axis coverage during a single, rapid rotation of the gantry coupled with optimized heart rate, pitch (speed at which the table moves through the scanner relative to the gantry rotation speed), and reconstruction sector angle insures adequate overlapping of data for reconstruction. Typical coverage prescribed for

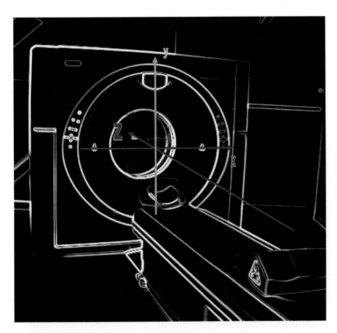

Figure 1.1 *Convention for labeling the x-, y-, and z-axes relative to the patient table (z-axis) and the scanner (x–y plane).*

cardiac imaging requires patient breath-hold of 10 to 12 seconds on current generation systems, which is feasible for most individuals including those with cardiovascular illness.

Adequate patient preparation cannot be overemphasized. This is a coordinated effort involving the scheduling staff, technologist, physician, and nurse. Documenting serum creatinine level and history of contrast allergy is essential at the time of scheduling. Just as with invasive angiography, the presence of renal insufficiency does not necessarily preclude cardiovascular multidetector CT (MDCT) examination; the risk of contrast nephropathy must be weighed against the benefit of the information to be gained from the procedure. If clinically indicated, some degree of renal protection may be achieved with pre- and postintravenous saline hydration. Some clinicians find a benefit to *N*-acetylcysteine administration as well. Similarly, eliciting a history of contrast allergy can prompt appropriate pretreatment to attenuate or prevent a contrast reaction in susceptible individuals if the risk is acceptable to both patient and referring clinician.

Even with the shortest effective gantry rotation times currently available, inadequate heart rate control can adversely affect image quality, particularly in the setting of a highly variable heart rate. Thus, the judicious use of medications to slow the heart rate, assuming appropriate screening for contraindications to such drugs, greatly increases the likelihood of having high-quality, motion artifact–free images for interpretation. Conversely, in the setting of atrial fibrillation or frequent ectopy rendering the heart rhythm highly irregular, administration of a vagolytic agent such as atropine may be appropriate; the irregularity of the cardiac rhythm has a more negative impact on image quality than increased heart rate alone. We seek to achieve a heart rate during scanning of ≤ 60 beats per minute, though higher heart rates with no variability such as those seen in the denervated post–cardiac transplant patient may also result in adequate image quality. Finally, the patient with a paced rhythm may warrant temporary reprogramming as tolerated to render the electrocardiographic trigger stable during scanning. Advances in multiple source scanner technology may ultimately improve temporal resolution to the point where heart rate is no longer a factor in cardiac CT.

The scan itself is performed with peripheral venous administration of iodinated contrast material. A small bolus of contrast (timing bolus) can be used to determine the delay between intravenous injection and the appearance of the bolus in the structure of interest, typically the ascending aorta for coronary imaging. This delay is then used in the volume acquisition. Alternatively, a Hounsfield unit (HU) threshold (measurement of x-ray attenuation) may be set such that once this threshold is reached in the structure of interest, the volume scan is triggered (bolus tracking). The advantage of bolus tracking is that the total volume administered is reduced, assuming that the technologists performing the procedure have facility in recognizing when to manually start the scan, if necessary. During the breath-hold acquisition, radiation dose can be minimized on the basis of variable x-ray attenuation in different sections of the body (e.g., less radiation needed in the neck vs. the mid-chest) or the electrocardiogram (ECG). Most systems now offer some form of ECG dose modulation such that less radiation is delivered during portions of the cardiac cycle with significant motion, and these are therefore less suitable for coronary reconstruction. A few ectopic beats during the acquisition can be edited

out during reformatting of the raw data if they result in significant artifact (Chapter 5) but are best dealt with *before* the scan with pharmacologic maneuvers or pacemaker reprogramming.

Once the raw data has been acquired, it is converted to thin axial images, with all current 64-detector scanner platforms providing submillimeter spatial resolution. Reformatting to thicker sections is helpful for maximum intensity projection (MIP) image review. When reviewing coronary artery segments with stents, one should review the thinnest sections possible, as well as images generated with both smooth and sharp reconstruction kernels (**Fig. 1.2**). Generating multiphase axial sections allows dynamic rendering of the volume or specific structures of interest.

All workstation platforms allow several image review modes including sequential review of the axial images, simultaneous MPR image review in axial/coronal/sagittal planes, volume rendering, and dynamic review of multiphase data. Many have advocated reviewing the entire data set from the axial plane. A complementary approach focused on the coronary arteries is to start from the axial plane in a three-dimensional MPR screen, identify and evaluate the left mainstem, then go through the entire coronary tree segment by segment [e.g., proximal left anterior descending coronary artery (LAD), mid-LAD, distal LAD, and diagonal branches] by optimizing the three imaging planes to visualize each segment. This insures that the entire coronary tree is evaluated but requires more user interaction to generate

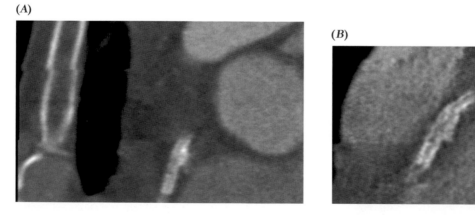

(A)

(B)

Figure 1.2 *(A) MPR image of an RCA stent generated using a soft (B20f, Siemens, Erlanger, Germany) reconstruction kernel. (B) Same RCA stent generated using a sharper (B46f) kernel demonstrates less blurring of the stent struts.*

(A)

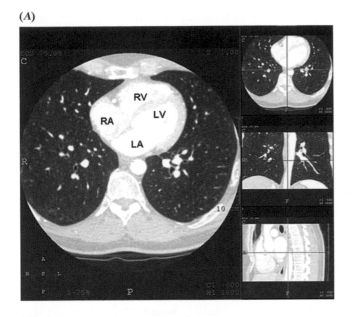

(B)

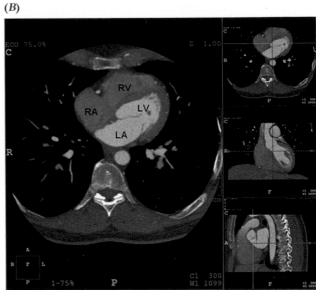

(C)

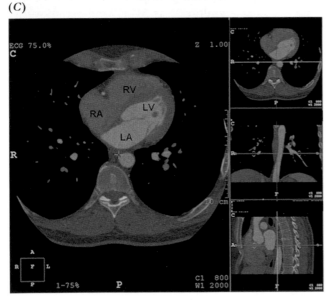

Figure 1.3   *Window width and window center are set by the user when reviewing CT images to optimize viewing of lung (**A**) center -600, width 1600 HU; contrast-filled structures (**B**), center 300, width 1099; and bone or high-attenuation structures, (**C**) center 800, width 2000 HU.*

adequate views of each segment. Technologists may become facile in generating thin maximum intensity projections in batches along the LAD, left circumflex coronary artery, and right coronary artery, which may further simplify coronary artery assessment but does not replace careful interrogation of each segment by the interpreting physician. Volume rendering is useful to gain an overview of graft anatomy in patients who have undergone coronary artery bypass surgery; surveying the ascending aorta is important to identify all grafts including those that may be occluded. Continued developments in image

segmentation make this an ever-evolving field; the individual practitioner should be thoroughly familiar with all of the available image review and segmentation techniques on their workstation platforms for those instances when the routine approach is insufficient to answer the clinical questions.

Window width and window center determine dynamic range and contrast when displaying CT images; adjusting window settings allows management of the breadth of signal intensity information captured in the range of HU such that particular structures or tissues are more easily appreciated. Thus, certain combinations are more suited for review of different regions as illustrated in **Figure 1.3**. Using a so-called lung window with window center of -600 HU and window width of 1600 HU, **Figure 1.3A** demonstrates optimal viewing of structures in the lung parenchyma. Moving the center to 300 HU improves visualization of contrast-filled structures, as seen in **Figure 1.3B**, and moving it still higher to a bone window centered around 800 HU (**Fig. 1.3C**) improves delineation of bony or high-attenuation structures.

Chapter 2 Normal cardiac anatomy

Anatomic considerations when reviewing cardiac computed tomography (CT) images can be classified into axial plane anatomy and cardiac plane anatomy. Serial sections from cranial to caudal are presented in **Figure 2.1. Figure 2.2** demonstrates the cardiac chambers as viewed from straight sagittal, coronal, and axial planes. From these default planes, one may adjust the axes of multiplanar reformatting to conform to the cardiac planes (**Fig. 2.3**). The short axis is defined as being orthogonal to the interventricular septum from apex (beyond distal insertion

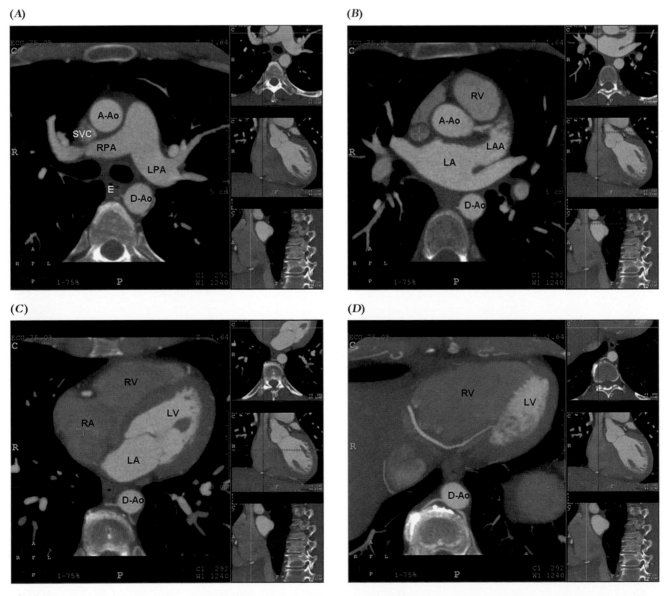

Figure 2.1 *Cranial to caudal (**A–D**) images obtained in the axial plane.* Abbreviations: *AAo, ascending aorta; DAo, descending aorta; E, esophagus; LA, left atrium; LAA, left atrial appendage; LPA, left pulmonary artery; LV, left ventricle; RA, right atrium; RPA, right pulmonary artery; RV, right ventricle; SVC, superior vena cava.*

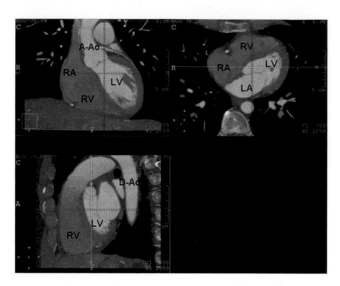

Figure 2.2 *Cardiac chambers, as viewed from straight coronal* (top left), *axial* (top right), *and sagittal* (bottom left) *planes.*

of the papillary muscles) to base (at the level of the mitral annulus). Cardiac planes are important to identify when reviewing segmental wall motion of the left ventricle (LV), as the standard LV segmentation nomenclature is based on the conventions defining these planes. From end-systolic and end-diastolic images (**Fig. 2.4**), one can compute ventricular volumes, ejection fraction, and myocardial mass. While standardized nomenclature has not yet been developed for segmentation of the right ventricle (RV), RV inflow and outflow planes (**Fig. 2.5**), allow analysis of right heart–specific questions, particularly those involving the tricuspid and pulmonic valves. More details on cardiac function are provided in Chapter 6.

(A)

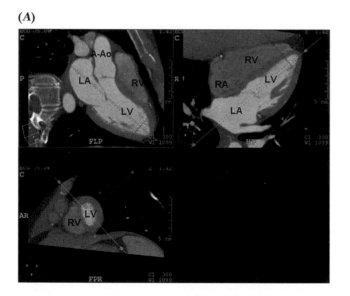

(B)

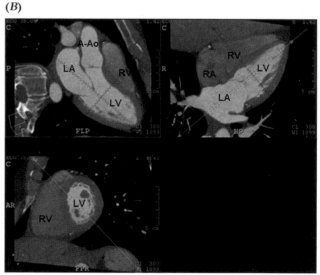

(C)

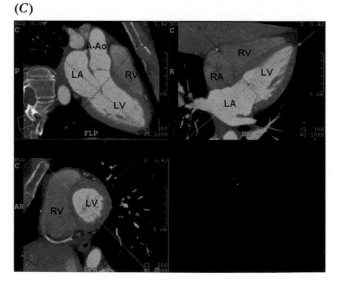

Figure 2.3 *Multiplanar reformatted images, keeping constant the three-chamber long axis* (top left) *and four-chamber or horizontal long-axis* (HLA, top right) *planes, while varying the short-axis plane from apex (**A**) to mid (**B**) and base (**C**), relative to the cardiac long-axis.*

(A)

(B)

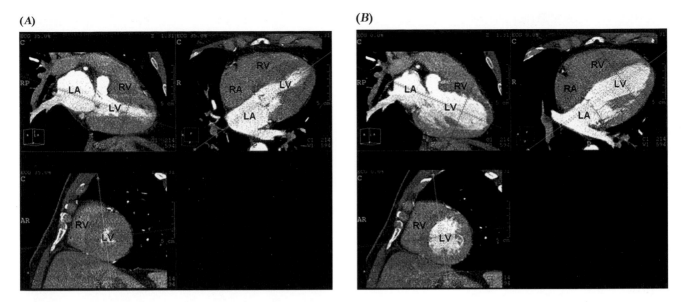

Figure 2.4 *Multiplanar reformatted images generated at the same spatial location but different cardiac phases: (**A**) end-systole and (**B**) end-diastole.*

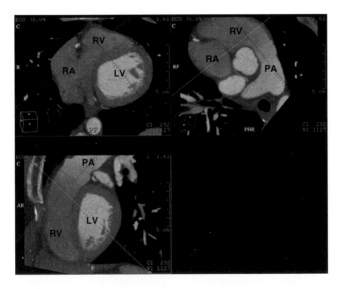

Figure 2.5 *Maximum intensity projections demonstrate various planes optimized to view right heart structures such as the right ventricular inflow tract (top left) and right ventricular outflow tract in oblique axial (top right) and sagittal (bottom left) planes.*

CORONARY ARTERIES

When reviewing coronary arteries, a typical first step is identifying the coronary artery ostia. This view helps identify coronary artery anomalies and ostial disease and is generated by moving along the aortic root parallel to the aortic valve (**Fig. 2.6**).

CLINICAL CASE 1

A 57-year-old Caucasian female with a 70 pack-year history of tobacco use, hyperlipidemia, and peripheral arterial disease presented for evaluation of chest pain. Nuclear stress testing demonstrated good functional capacity, exercising nine minutes of the Bruce protocol. Perfusion imaging indicated a mid-anterior wall defect (**Fig. 2.7**).

Coronary multidetector CT (MDCT) showed excellent visualization of the entire coronary tree, including the left anterior descending artery (LAD, **Fig. 2.8**), a small-diameter circumflex artery (**Fig. 2.9**), and the proximal and distal segments of the right coronary artery (**Figs. 2.10** and **2.11**), which was free of atherosclerotic disease.

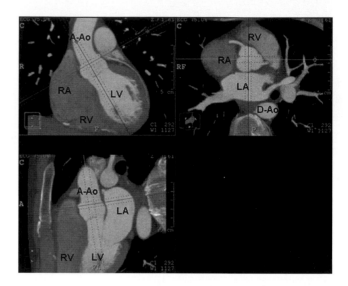

Figure 2.6 *Maximum intensity projections demonstrate the coronary ostia arising normally from the right and left sinuses of Valsalva. This plane* (top right) *is identified by moving along the aortic root parallel to the aortic valve, as shown in the corresponding oblique coronal* (top left) *and sagittal* (bottom left) *maximum intensity projection images.*

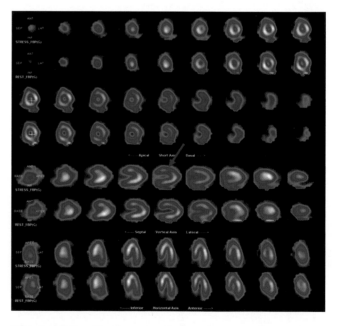

Figure 2.7 *Nuclear perfusion images demonstrate a reversible anterior perfusion defect versus breast attenuation artifact* (arrow).

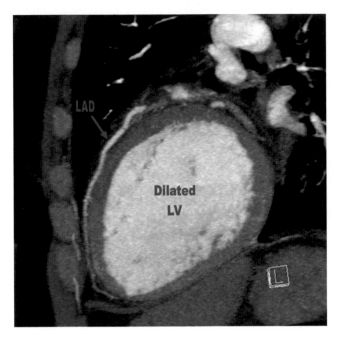

Figure 2.8 *Axial MIP image showing a normal LAD. Abbreviations: MIP, maximum intensity projection image; LAD, left anterior descending artery.*

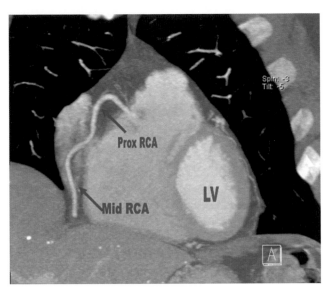

Figure 2.10 *Normal proximal and mid-portions of the right coronary artery* (arrows).

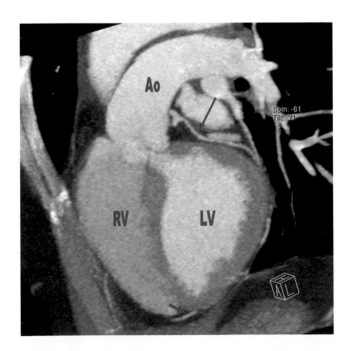

Figure 2.9 *Small, nondominant circumflex artery* (long arrow). *Note the small portion of the distal RCA is also visualized* (short arrow). Abbreviation: *RCA, right coronary artery.*

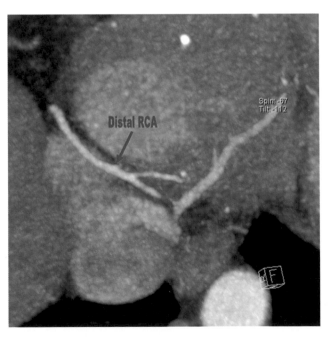

Figure 2.11 *Normal distal portion of the RCA* (arrow). Abbreviation: *RCA, right coronary artery.*

CLINICAL CASE 2

A 43-year-old African American female smoker with a history of shortness of breath presumed to be due to obstructive airway disease presented for evaluation of chest pain and dyspnea. The physical examination was notable for a laterally displaced left heart border by percussion. Cardiac CT angiography (CTA) was performed to assess for coronary disease.

Coronary CTA showed normal coronary arterial anatomy. Reformatted images (**Fig. 2.12**) showed LV dilatation. Calculated LV ejection fraction was 35%, consistent with nonischemic cardiomyopathy.

Cardiac catheterization confirmed global systolic dysfunction and normal coronary anatomy. In addition, invasive hemodynamics identified elevated left ventricular end-diastolic pressures consistent with diastolic dysfunction.

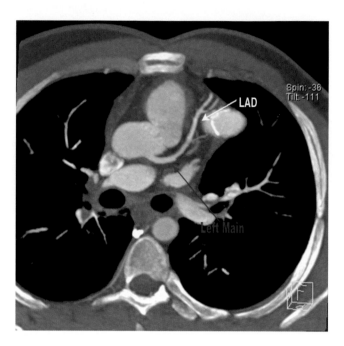

Figure 2.12 *Normal origin and course of the LAD, which is free of disease.* Abbreviations: *LV, left ventricle; LAD, left anterior descending artery.*

CLINICAL CASE 3

A 27-year-old Caucasian male with aortic coarctation presented for evaluation of coronary artery anatomy prior to surgical repair.

Coronary CTA demonstrated normal origin and proximal course of coronary arteries (**Fig. 2.13**). In addition, all segments of the coronary tree were well visualized and shown to be free of disease.

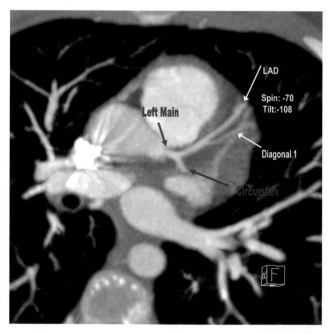

Figure 2.13 *The normal left main, LAD, diagonal and circumflex coronary arteries are seen.* Abbreviation: *LAD, left anterior descending artery.*

CLINICAL CASE 4

A 67-year-old male with hypertension and history of premature ventricular contractions (PVCs) presented for evaluation of increased frequency of PVCs with chest discomfort. The patient had invasive angiography five years ago that showed no obstructive disease but recalls that the procedure took longer than expected and wished to avoid recurrent invasive angiography if feasible. Coronary CTA was performed instead and showed posteriorly rotated ostium of the left coronary artery (**Fig. 2.14**). Coronary arteries were confirmed to be free of obstructive disease.

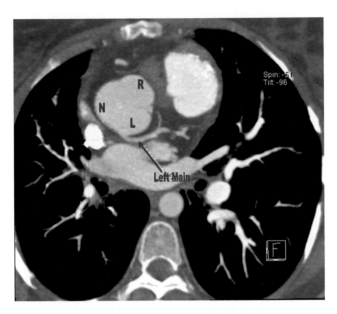

Figure 2.14 *Posteriorly rotated ostium* (arrow) *of the left coronary artery.* Abbreviations: *N, noncoronary; R, right; L, left coronary cusps.*

NORMAL CARDIAC CHAMBERS

CLINICAL CASE 5

A 48-year-old female with chest pain underwent stress testing that demonstrated electrocardiographic abnormalities with exercise but normal perfusion imaging. Due to persistent dyspnea, she was referred for cardiac CTA. Coronary arteries were free of disease. Multiplanar reformatted images (**Fig. 2.15**) showed normal cardiac chamber size. Cine CT demonstrated normal biventricular function.

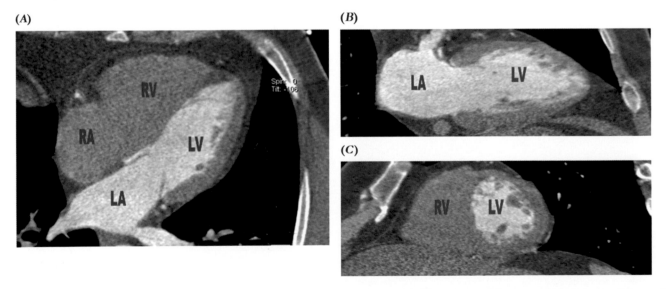

Figure 2.15 *Normal RA, RV, LA, and left ventricle in the horizontal long axis (**A**), vertical long axis (**B**), and short axis (**C**) views.* Abbreviations: *RA, right atrium; RV, right ventricle; LA, left atrium.*

VALVES

CLINICAL CASE 6

A 27-year-old male with a family history of premature CAD presented for evaluation of syncope. Transthoracic echocardiography showed normal systolic function and no significant valvular abnormalities. CTA showed normal coronary anatomy, normal LV systolic size and function, and excellent visualization of the valves, which were free of disease (**Figs. 2.16** and **2.17**).

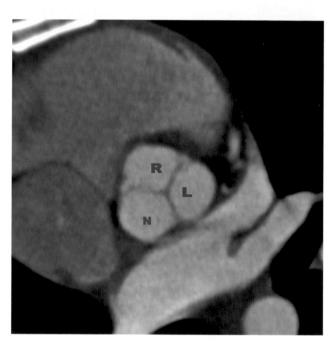

Figure 2.16 *Normal tri-leaflet aortic valve consisting of right (R), left (L), and noncoronary (N) cusps.*

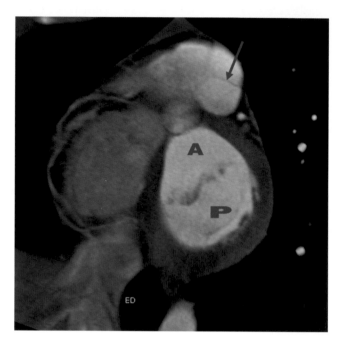

Figure 2.17 *Normal mitral valve consisting of anterior (A) and posterior (P) leaflets. Note that the pulmonic valve is also seen in this view* (arrow).

CLINICAL PEARLS

- CTA is important in assessing patients with equivocal stress imaging results. This is particularly true for female patients with breast tissue attenuation. These female patients can be quickly and less invasively evaluated by CTA to facilitate timely medical therapy and/or intervention.

- Patients who present with symptoms of congestive heart failure and clinical findings of left ventricular dysfunction can be evaluated by CTA. Both the left ventricular function and the coronary tree can be assessed, helping determine the etiology of the left ventricular dysfunction.

- Patients who have had untoward clinical experiences with cardiac catheterization or have had recent cardiac interventions and refuse repeat cardiac catheterization can successfully be evaluated by noninvasive CT coronary angiography.

- CTA allows excellent visualization of cardiac valves, with appropriate reformatting to generate *en face* views. Left heart valves are better seen than right heart valves on routine coronary CTA studies due to concentration of contrast in the LV and aorta.

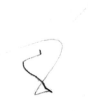

Chapter 3   Abnormal coronary arteries

Before analyzing the cases in this chapter, it is helpful to consider the optimal protocols for coronary imaging, how to analyze diseased coronaries, how to evaluate plaques, and how to recognize and avoid artifacts.

The key to obtaining optimal coronary computed tomography angiography (CTA) images is timing: timing of the heart rate, timing of the contrast delivery during the scan, and timing of the scan itself with respect to the latter two. Careful attention must be given to lower the heart rate to 50 to 60 BPM prior to the scan. This allows for the optimal reduction of artifact induced by coronary and myocardial motion during the scan.

Optimal contrast delivery during the scan requires an appreciation for the time it takes for the contrast to travel from the intravenous injection site to the site of interest, e.g., the proximal aorta for coronary artery studies. This can be estimated using a timing bolus scan, during which a single axial location is repeatedly imaged after injection of a low volume of contrast (e.g., 20 cc). The resulting images allow graphical display of the signal intensity versus time and measurement of the delay (seconds) to peak signal intensity in the aortic root. This delay is then used during the volume acquisition with the full contrast load. Alternatively, bolus tracking available on most scanners allows setting of a Hounsfield unit (HU) threshold (e.g., 100) in a region of interest in a specific image location such as the aortic root. In bolus tracking, an additional timing bolus scan is not required; rather, the volume acquisition is triggered during a premonitoring phase once the threshold HU level is reached in the region of interest.

The patient must hold their breath during the scan. Reviewing the importance of following breathhold instructions with the patient prior to placing them in the scanner coupled with observation of breathhold compliance during timing bolus scan (if used) gives one the best opportunity to assure good breathholding during the volume acquisition. Respiratory artifact is obvious when reviewing the thin sections reconstructed in a nonaxial plane (see Chapter 5: Artifacts) and does not lend itself well to postprocessing editing techniques; it is much better avoided with patient understanding and cooperation, if feasible.

The acquisition technique requires slight modifications when assessing patients with coronary artery bypass grafts (CABG). It can be disheartening to review the images after the fact, seeing bypass grafts and not their proximal origins because the history of bypass surgery was not appreciated by the person scanning. Multiple levels of inquiry, e.g., at the time of scheduling and by the person screening the patient preprocedure asking if the patient has every undergone bypass surgery help avoid this situation. Recognition of sternotomy wires on topograms should also prompt further inquiry into bypass surgery history if not already known. In addition to increased volume of coverage to include the proximal anastomosis (we prescribe the scan to start above the subclavian arteries on all CABG cases), the delay between initiating contrast injection and scanning should be shorter since there is a greater volume to cover. With timing bolus delay programming, we typically shorten the delay by four seconds, and, with bolus tracking, we keep the ROI in the aortic root but lower the HU threshold to 80 to trigger scanning earlier.

Image analysis requires reconstruction of the raw data to generate thin axial sections that can be reviewed and analyzed using any of a number of rendering techniques. We choose to generate these thin sections at multiple phases of the cardiac cycle, because some segments of the coronary tree may be blurred at one phase but more stationary, and therefore more interpretable, at a different phase. The optimal phase may differ from one segment to another, underscoring the need to have thin sections generated across multiple phases for review. By starting at the coronary artery ostia and systematically marching down each segment of the coronary tree and branches, including left mainstem, left anterior descending artery (LAD), left circumflex artery, and right coronary artery (RCA), one is assured of assessing each segment for disease. Some authors advocate image review in the axial plane, which is certainly an important component of overall image interpretation but may be insufficient for disease recognition and severity assessment. Starting from the coronary ostia, which typically have the largest caliber with gradual tapering of the vessels toward the distal segments, allows one to be attuned to abrupt changes in vessel appearance. The multitude of software packages available for coronary CTA image analysis precludes summary in this text, though all have the multiple tools needed for image review, i.e., multiplanar reconstructions, maximum intensity projections (MIPs), volume rendering, etc.

Recognizing artifact remains an important component of coronary CTA image review, despite advances in technology. Viewing the whole heart in a sagittal or coronal reformatted plane allows recognition of "stair-step" or "zipper-like" artifact due to chest wall motion. Artifact due to cardiac motion can be recognized with the multiphase image analysis, toggling between thin sections at various cardiac phases at sites of suspected disease. Some scanner platforms allow manual editing of the reconstruction to eliminate contribution of data acquired during ectopic beats; this can be very helpful when there are a few, isolated ectopic beats. Suspected lesions on CTA can be assessed from multiple projections, as well as in cross-section with semi-automatic segmentation of the vessel along its length or by manually generating a plane that shows the segment of interest in cross-section.

It may be obvious to state that avoiding artifact is preferred to trying to interpret around artifact whenever possible. Patient instruction and rhythm management have already been discussed. Not all artifacts, particularly those due to implanted devices, can be completely avoided and warrant acknowledgment in the report when trying to make conclusions about the presence and severity of coronary artery pathology. A typical example is the assessment of the RCA in the presence of right heart pacemaker or defibrillator leads. Unanticipated jumps in heart rate due to the patient's response to contrast infusion may also occur but are minimized with patient preparation that may include beta-blocker medications. It cannot be overemphasized that the time invested by the staff before the scan to optimize heart rate, acquisition timing, and breathholding facilitates interpretation of the resulting images to deliver the necessary clinical information.

CALCIFICATION

CLINICAL CASE 1

A 45-year-old male with hypertension, hyperlipidemia, and family history of premature CAD presented for evaluation of intermittent chest and right arm pain, not reliably precipitated by exertion. Physical examination and resting electrocardiography were unremarkable.

After initial cardiac enzymes showed no evidence of acute coronary syndrome, the patient underwent stress testing. At five minutes of exercise on the Bruce protocol, he developed ST segment depression and transient chest discomfort. Coronary CTA was rapidly completed and showed severe obstructive disease in the proximal LAD, proximal left circumflex, and RCA (**Figs. 3.1–3.3**). Invasive angiography confirmed high-grade coronary stenoses (**Fig. 3.4**). Both CTA and invasive catheterization (**Figs. 3.5** and **3.6**, respectively) demonstrated patency of the internal mammary arteries, which were subsequently used for surgical revascularization.

Role of CTA: 64-slice CTA readily identified both the calcified plaque and the adjacent low-attenuation noncalcified plaque. In this case, it provided a guide to further management of a patient with risk factors but inconclusive symptoms and resting parameters. This could potentially have been performed instead of stress testing, rather than in addition to stress testing, preventing potential risk due to exercise in the setting of high-grade coronary stenosis. Excellent visualization of the lesion and the entire coronary tree could be sufficient to proceed directly to intervention, rather than requiring repeat catheter-based diagnostic angiography.

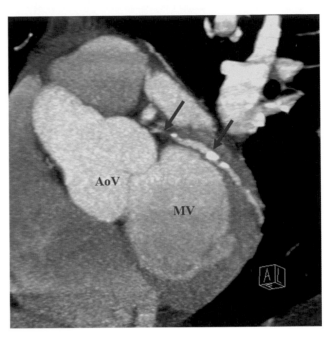

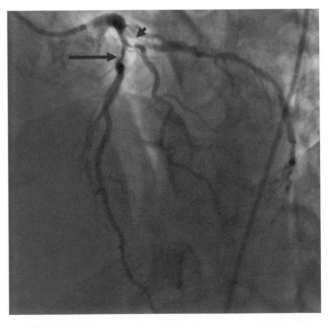

Figure 3.1 *High-grade obstructive lesion in the proximal LAD* (arrow). *Note the relative low attenuation consistent with noncalcified plaque. Serial calcified plaque is seen in the mid-LAD distal to this stenosis.* Abbreviations: *AAo, ascending aorta; LA, left atrium; RVOT, right ventricular outflow tract; LAD, left anterior descending artery.*

Figure 3.3 *An oblique left lateral view demonstrating serial disease in the left circumflex coronary artery* (arrows). Abbreviations: *AoV, aortic valve; MV, mitral valve inflow.*

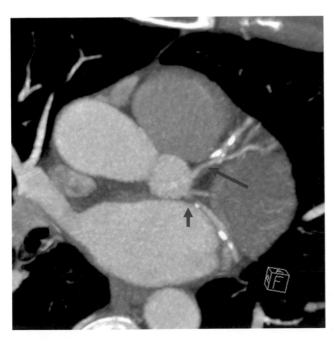

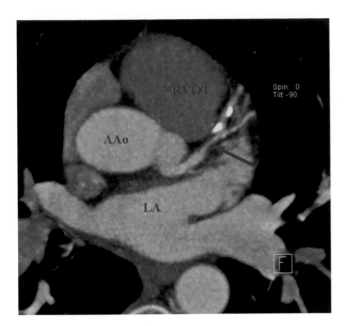

Figure 3.2 *Obstructive coronary artery disease is demonstrated in the LAD* (arrow) *and circumflex arteries* (small arrow). Abbreviation: *LAD, left anterior descending artery.*

Figure 3.4 *Invasive angiogram of the left coronary artery showing high-grade stenoses in the LAD* (arrow) *and LCx* (arrowhead). Abbreviations: *LAD, left anterior descending artery; LCx, left circumflex coronary artery.*

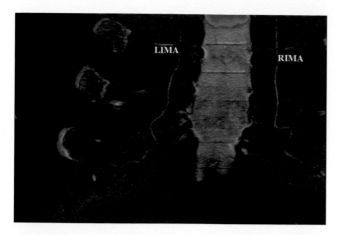

Figure 3.5 *Normal LIMA and RIMA bilaterally seen in the native positions along the sternum, demonstrating that these vessels are suitable for use as conduits for surgical revascularization.* Abbreviations: *LIMA, left internal mammary artery; RIMA, right internal mammary artery.*

CLINICAL CASE 2

A 26-year-old male smoker with diabetes, cocaine use, and family history of CAD presented for evaluation of chest pain and syncope. Physical examination revealed no evidence of structural heart disease or orthostasis. Stress nuclear imaging was negative for ischemia. Cardiac magnetic resonance imaging showed normal left ventricle (LV) size and systolic function, LV ejection fraction (EF) 65%, normal dimensions of thoracic and abdominal aorta, and no ischemia with dobutamine infusion (**Fig. 3.7**).

Because of clinical concern for subclinical atherosclerosis, the patient subsequently underwent coronary CTA that identified focal calcific plaque in proximal LAD obscuring luminal assessment (**Fig. 3.8**).

Role of CTA: CTA, in this case, made the diagnosis of coronary atherosclerosis, which would have gone undetected with stress testing alone in this relatively young patient.

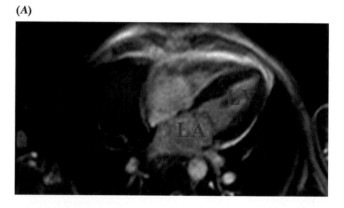

(A)

(B)

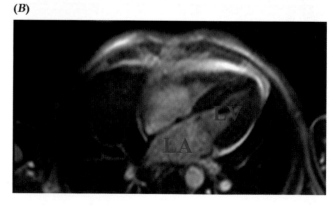

Figure 3.6 *Patent left internal mammary artery by selective invasive angiography.* Abbreviations: *SC, subclavian artery; LIMA, left internal mammary artery.*

Figure 3.7 *Rest (**A**) and stress (**B**) end-systolic frames of cine CMR imaging in the horizontal long axis plane show appropriate augmentation of LV contractility with inotropic stress.* Abbreviations: *LA, left atrium; LV, left ventricle.*

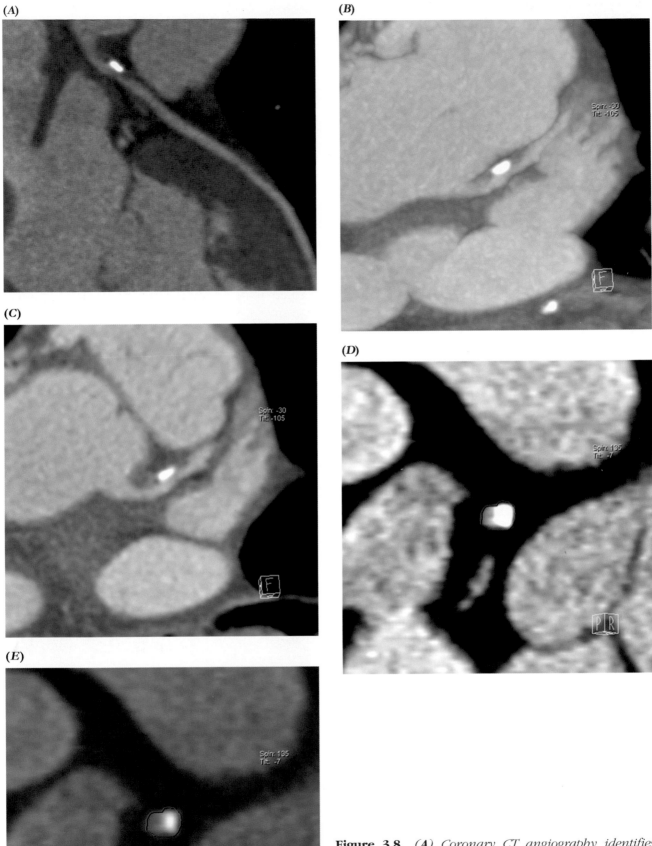

Figure 3.8 (**A**) *Coronary CT angiography identifies focal calcification in the proximal LAD.* (**B**) *A maximum intensity projection image, slice thickness 5 mm, worsens bloom artifact. This is reduced by reviewing this vessel segment as a thin multiplanar reformatted image (0.75 mm,* **C**). *Window width and level settings can also be adjusted to facilitate assessment of luminal stenosis at calcified sites (**D**: W406; **C**: 293; **E**: W1402, C458).* Abbreviation: *LAD, left anterior descending artery.*

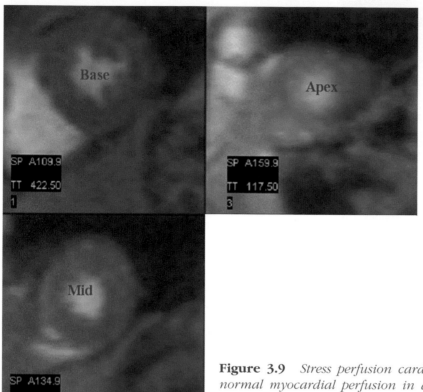

Figure 3.9   *Stress perfusion cardiac magnetic resonance demonstrates normal myocardial perfusion in all basal, mid-, and apical short axis segments.*

CLINICAL CASE 3

A 73-year-old male with hypertension and hyperlipidema presented for evaluation of vague atypical chest discomfort. Multiple prior stress tests demonstrated stress-induced ischemic electrocardiographic changes, though stress wall motion and perfusion had always been normal. Most recently, stress perfusion cardiac magnetic resonance (CMR) had also been completely normal (**Fig. 3.9**). Coronary CTA showed extensive calcification in the coronaries, indicating the presence of atherosclerosis (**Figs. 3.10** and **3.11**).

Role of CTA: CTA was able to detect diffuse atherosclerosis in this patient's coronary arteries, whereas stress testing revealed lack of functional compromise. The establishment of coronary atherosclerosis is key in this patient to be able to institute secondary prevention therapies that otherwise might not be utilized.

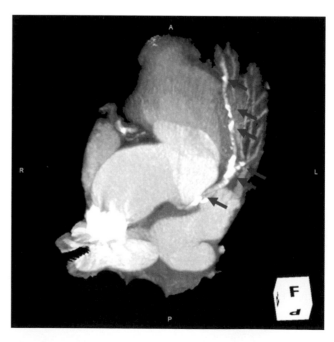

Figure 3.10   *Serial calcific atherosclerosis in the left coronary artery obscuring luminal assessment* (arrows).

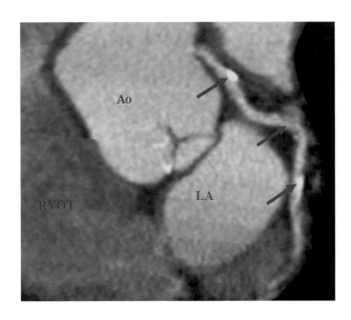

Figure 3.11 *Serial atherosclerotic plaque in the circumflex coronary artery* (arrows). *Abbreviations: Ao, aorta, LA, left atrium; RVOT, right ventricular outflow tract.*

NONCALCIFIED PLAQUE

CLINICAL CASE 4

A 37-year-old obese male with diabetes, hypertension, hypercholesterolemia, and family history of coronary artery disease (CAD) presented for evaluation of episodic, sharp, midsternal chest pain.

After cardiac enzymes showed no evidence of acute coronary syndrome, he underwent nuclear stress testing. After exercising 8.3 minutes of the Bruce protocol, he stopped due to shortness of breath and prior to achieving target heart rate, resulting in nuclear images that showed no ischemia at the heart rate achieved.

To better define the presence or absence of atherosclerosis, he was referred for coronary CTA. This showed soft plaque in the mid-LAD without significant luminal obstruction (**Fig. 3.12**). There was no disease identified in the RCA (**Fig. 3.13**). Cardiac catheterization confirmed isolated plaque disease (**Fig. 3.14**) as well as diastolic dysfunction of the LV.

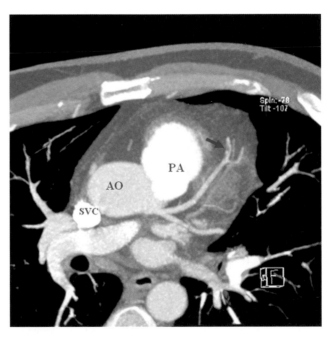

Figure 3.12 *Soft plaque in the distal LAD* (arrow). *Note suboptimal contrast timing, with greater concentration of contrast in the PA compared to the AO, indicating premature image acquisition. Abbreviations: SVC, superior vena cava; AO; ascending aorta; PA, pulmonary artery; LAD, left anterior descending artery.*

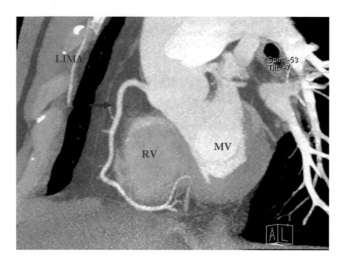

Figure 3.13 *Excellent visualization of the entire right coronary artery with CT angiography* (arrow). *Note that a portion of the LIMA is also seen in this plane.* Abbreviations: *RV, right ventricle; MV, mitral valve; LIMA, left internal mammary artery.*

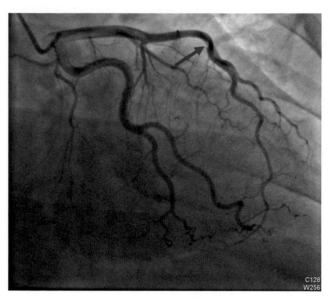

Figure 3.14 *Invasive coronary angiography/ lumenography shows mild luminal irregularity in the LAD, suggestive of nonobstructive plaque.* Abbreviation: *LIMA, left internal mammary artery.*

CLINICAL CASE 5

A 68-year-old female smoker with hyperlipidemia presented for coronary CTA. This demonstrated both calcified and noncalcified plaque in the coronary arteries (**Figs. 3.15** and **3.16**).

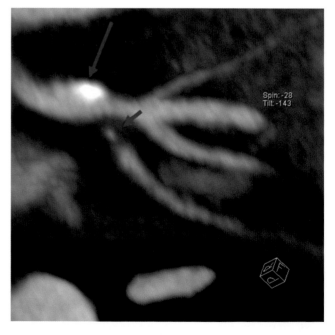

Figure 3.15 *Coronary CTA demonstrates both nonobstructive calcified plaque* (arrow) *and obstructive soft plaque in the circumflex coronary artery* (short arrow).

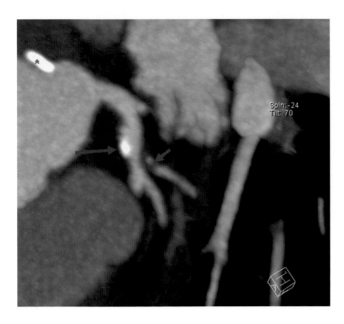

Figure 3.16 *Calcified plaque in the proximal left circumflex artery* (arrow) *and soft plaque at the ostium of a subtotally occluded OM branch* (short arrow). *Also note the calcification in the aortic root* (*). Abbreviation: *OM, obtuse marginal.*

CLINICAL CASE 6

A 63-year-old male with type 2 diabetes mellitus, hyperlipidemia, and hypertension presented for evaluation of fatigue and intermittent chest pain. Stress testing demonstrated fair exercise tolerance and ischemic ST depression. Sestamibi images were negative for ischemia.

Coronary CTA showed high-grade stenosis in the mid-circumflex artery due to lipid plaque with outward vessel remodeling at the site of stenosis (**Fig. 3.17**), as well as significant lipid plaque in proximal LAD (**Fig. 3.18**) without significant luminal narrowing. This outward, or positive, vessel wall remodeling is termed the "Glagov phenomenon" and is associated with increased risk of plaque rupture.

Cardiac catheterization confirmed high-grade stenosis in left circumflex coronary artery (LCx) and plaque disease in the proximal LAD (**Fig. 3.19**). He subsequently underwent successful percutaneous coronary angioplasty and stent placement at the site of LCx stenosis. At one-year follow-up, repeat coronary CTA demonstrated patency of the LCx stent (**Fig. 3.20**).

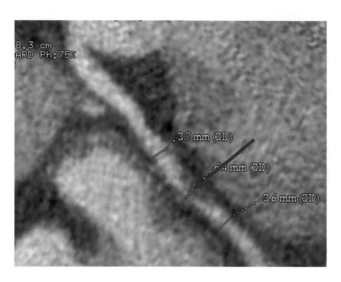

Figure 3.17 *Severe stenosis in the proximal LCx (arrow) with positive vessel wall remodeling; note the increased vessel diameter at the site of stenosis (6.4 mm) compared to the adjacent vessel segments (3.6–3.7 mm).* Abbreviation: *LCx, left circumflex coronary artery.*

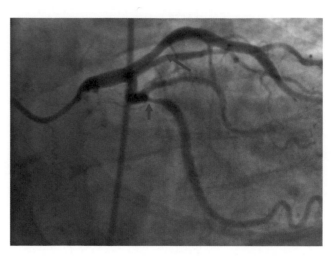

Figure 3.19 *Invasive angiogram confirming high-grade stenosis of the LCx* (short arrow) *and mild luminal irregularity suggestive of plaque in the proximal LAD* (arrow). Abbreviations: *LAD, left anterior descending artery; LCx, left circumflex coronary artery.*

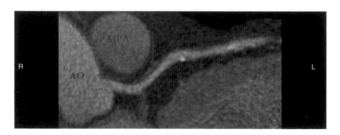

Figure 3.18 *Nonobstructive soft plaque in the proximal LAD* (arrow). Abbreviations: *MPA, main pulmonary artery; AO, ascending aorta; LAD, left anterior descending artery.*

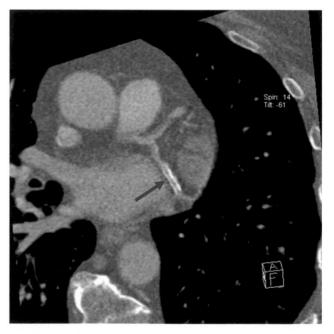

Figure 3.20 *Follow-up coronary CTA after one year demonstrates patency of the LCx stent* (arrow). Abbreviation: *LCx, left circumflex coronary artery.*

CLINICAL CASE 7

A 67-year-old male with diabetes, chronic lung disease, hypertension, and CAD with prior bypass surgery [left internal mammary artery (LIMA) to LAD, sequential saphenous vein graft (SVG) to diagonal and Ramus Intermedius branches of the left coronary artery] presented for evaluation of chest pain.

CTA showed high-grade stenosis at the ostium of the sequential SVG (**Fig. 3.21**). This was confirmed with invasive angiography (**Fig. 3.22**).

Role of CTA: In this patient with a history of coronary artery bypass surgery, deconditioning and lung disease would limit the feasibility of stress testing. CTA provided rapid, accurate non-invasive assessment of graft status.

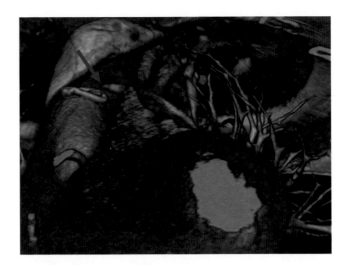

Figure 3.21 *Volume rendering of the CTA data demonstrates a high-grade ostial stenosis of a sequential SVG at the aortic anastomosis (arrow). Abbreviation: SVG, saphenous vein graft.*

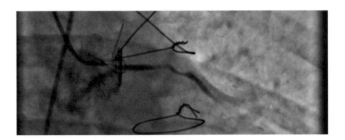

Figure 3.22 *Cardiac catheterization confirmed high-grade stenosis at the aortic anastomosis of a vein graft by both angiography (arrow) and abnormal contrast reflux, indicating ostial disease (short arrow).*

CLINICAL CASE 8

A 74-year-old male with hypertension and prior bypass surgery for CAD presented for evaluation of intermittent chest pain that was somewhat dissimilar from previous anginal episodes. CMR showed significant ischemia in the LAD distribution with vasodilator stress (**Fig. 3.23**). CTA showed a patent SVG to distal RCA (**Fig. 3.24**), patent SVG to obtuse marginal (OM) branch (**Fig. 3.25**), occluded SVG to diagonal branch (**Fig. 3.26**), and ostial stenosis at the aortic anastomosis of the SVG to distal LAD (**Fig. 3.27**).

Role of CTA: While stress perfusion CMR was helpful in confirming that myocardial ischemia was a potential mechanism for this patient's symptoms, CTA demonstrated a potential target for revascularization, namely, the ostial SVG stenosis. In this case, CTA was complementary to the functional information provided by CMR.

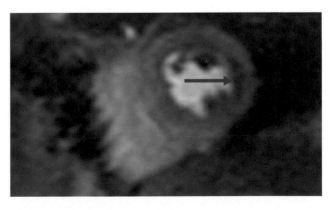

Figure 3.23 *Stress cardiac magnetic resonance perfusion images demonstrate ischemia in the LAD territory, particularly the anterolateral myocardium (arrow) and papillary muscle (*). Abbreviation: LAD, left anterior descending artery.*

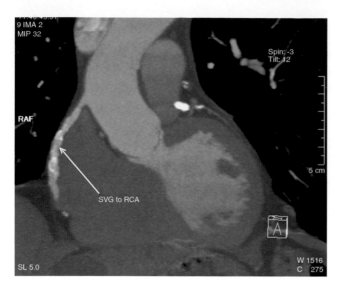

Figure 3.24 *Patent but diseased SVG to the RCA. Abbreviations: SVG, saphenous vein graft; RCA, right coronary artery.*

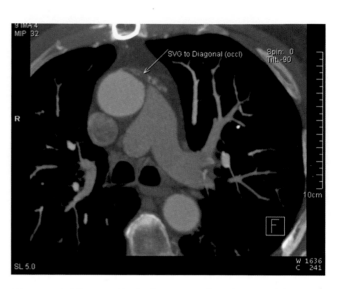

Figure 3.26 *Occluded SVG to the diagonal branch of the LAD. Abbreviations: SVG, saphenous vein graft; LAD, left anterior descending artery.*

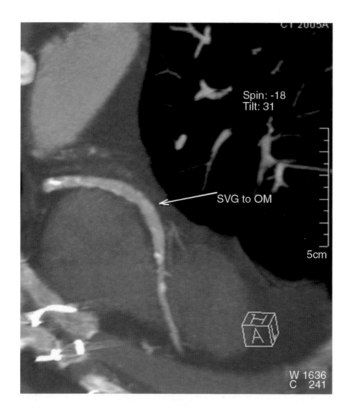

Figure 3.25 *Patent SVG to OM branch of the left circumflex coronary artery. Abbreviations: SVG, saphenous vein graft; OM, obtuse marginal.*

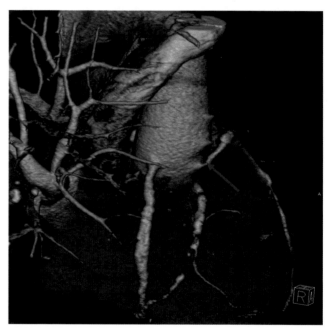

Figure 3.27 *Ostial stenosis at the aortic anastomosis of a saphenous vein graft to the left anterior descending artery (arrow).*

CLINICAL CASE 9

A 75-year-old male with diabetes, hypertension, hyperlipidemia, obesity, peripheral arterial disease, dementia, and prior coronary artery bypass surgery presented for evaluation of angina. He could not recall where he had undergone surgery, precluding review of the surgical history. Physical examination was significant for diminished right femoral and right dorsalis pedis pulses.

Stress electrocardiogram (ECG) was indeterminate due to baseline abnormalities; nuclear perfusion showed fixed anterior, apical, and inferior defects.

CTA showed a patent left internal mammary artery graft to the mid-LAD (**Figs. 3.28** and **3.29**) as well as a patent Ramus Intermedius limb of a sequential SVG (**Fig. 3.30**). The SVG sequence to an OM branch was occluded (**Fig. 3.30**).

Role of CTA: The advantage of CTA in this case in comparison to traditional catheter-based angiography is the ability to delineate the anastomosis of the grafts to the native coronaries with tissue and lumen detail without multiple catheter manipulations and contrast injections to identify occluded grafts. Lacking a target for repeat revascularization in the setting of fixed perfusion abnormalities, this patient was managed medically without requiring invasive angiography.

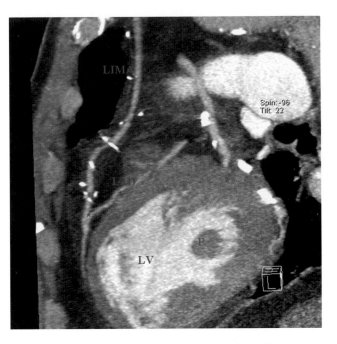

Figure 3.28 *Patent LIMA conduit to the left anterior descending coronary artery. Note excellent visualization of the distal anastomosis (*). Abbreviations: LV, left ventricle; P, hypertrophied papillary muscle; LIMA, left internal mammary artery.*

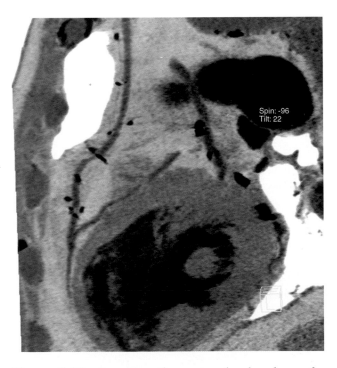

Figure 3.29 *Inverting the grayscale also shows the patent LIMA to LAD. Abbreviations: LIMA, left internal mammary artery; LAD, left anterior descending artery.*

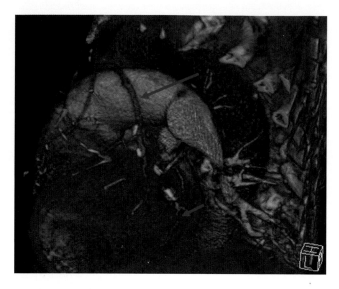

Figure 3.30 *Sequential SVG with patent limb to Ramus Intermedius* (arrow) *but occluded limb to an obtuse marginal* (short arrow). *Note the presence of surgical clips (*) but no contrast-filled lumen, indicating graft occlusion of the sequence limb.* Abbreviation: *SVG, saphenous vein graft.*

CLINICAL CASE 10

A 59 year-old male with CAD and prior bypass surgery presented for evaluation of syncope. CTA showed patent free radial graft to an OM branch of the circumflex coronary artery; however, the LIMA was not visualized, suggestive of occlusion (**Fig. 3.31**). Cardiac catheterization confirmed occlusion of the LIMA. Knowing the right internal mammary artery (RIMA) was patent (**Fig. 3.31**), he underwent repeat bypass surgery using this vessel as a conduit.

Role of CTA: Three-dimensional (3-D) CTA reformatting allows visualization of all opacified vessels within the scan volume; in this case, both the LIMA and RIMA should have been opacified. The free radial graft and native RIMA are visualized well, but careful search through the imaged volume showed no evidence of a contrast-filled LIMA. Nonopacification by CTA indicated occlusion, which was confirmed by conventional invasive angiography. This helped avoid a prolonged "hunt" for the LIMA with catheter-based angiography and also identified a patent arterial conduit (the RIMA) for use during repeat revascularization.

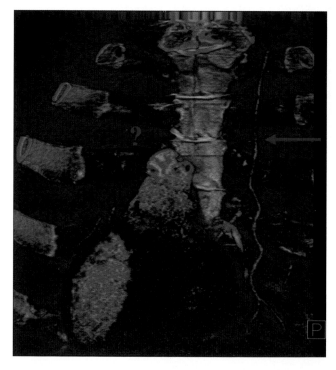

Figure 3.31 *A posterior view of the CTA data demonstrates that absence of a contrast-filled structure where the LIMA would usually lie (?), unlike the native RIMA that is well visualized* (arrow). Abbreviations: *LIMA, left internal mammary artery; RIMA, left internal mammary artery.*

STENTS

CLINICAL CASE 11

A 70-year-old female with diabetes, hypertension, hyperlipidemia, obesity, cerebrovascular disease, and CAD had previously undergone coronary artery stent placement (**Figs. 3.32** and **3.33**). Catheterization at that time had shown mild aortic valve stenosis. She returned three months later with dyspnea, fatigue, and peripheral edema and was referred for CTA examination.

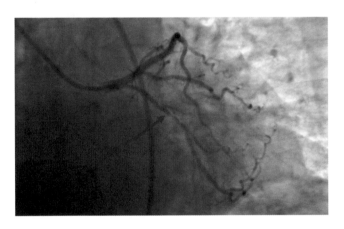

Figure 3.32 *Invasive angiogram three months prior to presentation shows severe stenosis of the OM branch of the circumflex artery* (arrow). Abbreviation: *OM, obtuse marginal.*

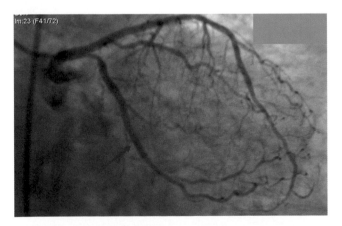

Figure 3.33 *Poststent angiogram shows restoration of obtuse marginal vessel caliber* (arrow) *after percutaneous intervention.*

CTA showed patent stents in the left anterior descending and obtuse marginal coronary arteries (**Fig. 3.34**), as well as a planimetered aortic valve area of 1.1 cm^2, consistent with stable, mild aortic stenosis.

Role of CTA: Evaluation of stents with CTA can be challenging due to blooming artifact that varies in severity on the basis of stent material, strut thickness, and reconstruction kernel (less blooming with sharper reconstruction kernels). Also, stents in small-diameter coronary segments may be difficult to assess. However, given the increasing use of stents and percutaneous coronary intervention to treat CAD, it is important to have reliable methods for noninvasive assessment of stent patency. CTA techniques to improve coronary stent assessment include review of multiplanar reformatted image instead of MIP images, generating thin sections with sharper reconstruction kernels that reduce blooming artifact, and careful interrogation of not only the lumen within the stent but also the coronary artery just proximal and distal to the stent margins.

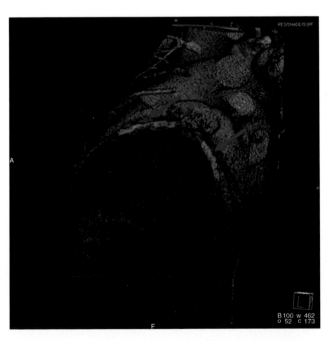

Figure 3.34 *Volume rendering of the heart, demonstrating stents in the LAD and LCx/OM coronary arteries* (arrows). Abbreviations: *LAD, left anterior descending artery; OM, obtuse marginal; LCx, left circumflex coronary artery.*

CLINICAL CASE 12

An 81-year-old male with hyperlipidemia, hypertension, history of inferior myocardial infarction (MI), and RCA stent placement presented for evaluation of nonexertional, sharp chest pain.

CTA showed patency of the RCA stents, both along its length (**Figs. 3.35** and **3.37**) and in cross-section (**Fig. 3.36**).

Role of CTA: The curved reformatting capacity allows the "uncurving" of a vessel in order to index the narrowest and widest portions of the vessel caliber to each other. In this case, it facilitates visualization of contrast-filling defects within the stented segment. It also allows "en face" evaluation of the length of the stented segment for the lack/presence of contrast.

(A)

(B)

Figure 3.35 *Length-wise rendering of the RCA with its proximal (pRCA) stent (**A**). Cross-section for Figure 35 is obtained from the planes outlined in (**B**). Good contrast opacification throughout the stent as well as the distal vessel are consistent with stent patency in this case.* Abbreviations: *RCA, right coronary artery; mRCA, mid-RCA.*

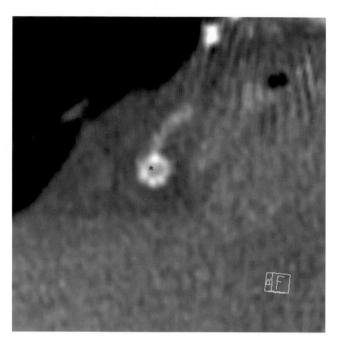

Figure 3.36 *Cross-sectional image of the RCA stent. Note: * denotes intrastent lumen.*

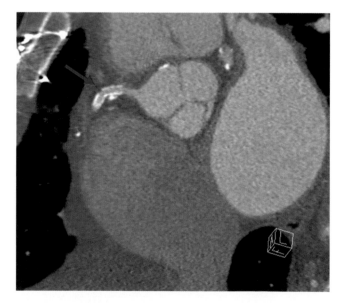

Figure 3.37 *Curved reformatted image demonstrates mild tortuosity in the proximal portion of the patent stent* (arrow).

CLINICAL CASE 13

A 68-year-old female smoker with diabetes, hypertension, and obesity presented for evaluation of chest pain in the setting of known CAD and prior percutaneous intervention.

CTA showed patency of a stent in the first obtuse marginal of the circumflex coronary artery (**Fig. 3.38**).

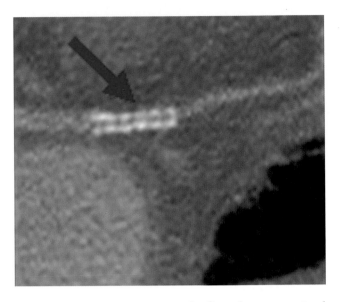

Figure 3.38   *Patent stent in the first obtuse marginal branch of the circumflex coronary artery* (arrow).

CLINICAL CASE 14

A 74-year-old female with hypertension, hyperlipidemia, and CAD status post circumflex artery stent placement presented for chest pain evaluation.

CTA showed patency of the proximal circumflex artery stent (**Fig. 3.39**).

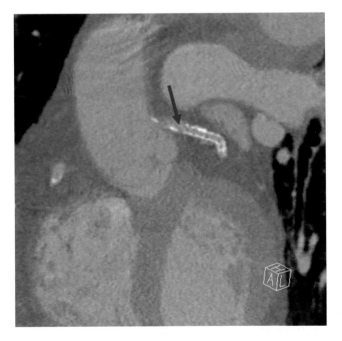

Figure 3.39   *Patent proximal left circumflex coronary artery stent* (arrow).

CORONARY ARTERY ECTASIA

CLINICAL CASE 15

A 58-year-old male with an implantable cardiac defibrillator for ventricular tachycardia presented for evaluation of dyspnea.

Cardiac catheterization one year prior to the current presentation demonstrated coronary artery ectasia (**Fig. 3.40**), defined as dilatation to at least 1.5 times that of an adjacent normal reference segment. There was hemodynamic evidence of diastolic dysfunction, manifest as elevated left ventricular end-diastolic pressure.

Repeat coronary assessment was performed with CTA to exclude progression of CAD as the cause of dyspnea. The study demonstrated ectasia of the coronary arteries (**Fig. 3.41**), prompting more aggressive medical management of known diastolic dysfunction.

Role of CTA: CTA 3-D reformatting allowed reproducible evaluation of the extent and caliber of ectasia in a patient in whom the pathology was known but serial assessment was needed. CTA provided this information noninvasively.

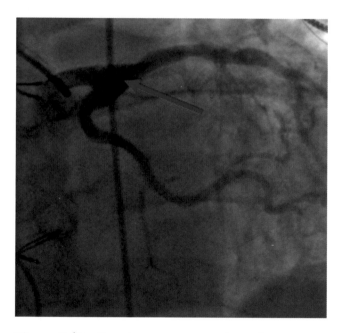

Figure 3.40 *Invasive coronary angiography one year prior to the current presentation shows ectasia, or non-obstructive dilatation of the left coronary artery* (arrow).

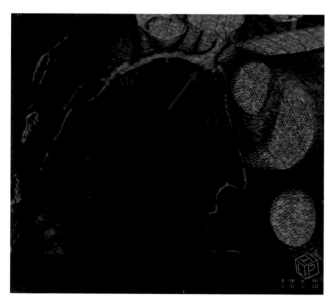

Figure 3.41 *Ectasia of the left coronary artery tree is most prominent at the bifurcation* (arrow) *into the left anterior descending arteries (LADs) and circumflex (LCx) arteries.*

CLINICAL CASE 16

A 56-year-old former smoker with diabetes, hyperlipidemia, hypertension, and a family history of CAD presented for cardiovascular assessment. He denied symptoms, though his wife remarked that he seemed more fatigued after a round of golf in recent months.

To assess for CAD, his internist referred him for coronary CTA. This demonstrated marked dilatation of the proximal coronary arteries and an abrupt decrease in coronary artery caliber in the postaneurysmal segments (**Figs. 3.42** and **3.43**). Both LIMA and RIMA were widely patent, and LV size and systolic function were normal: LVEDV 84 mL, LVESV 29 mL, EF 65%.

Invasive coronary angiography confirmed the presence of coronary artery aneurysms (**Fig. 3.44**). He subsequently underwent successful surgical revascularization using the internal mammary arteries as conduits.

Role of CTA: CTA demonstrated the presence of both coronary artery aneurysmal dilatation and discrete stenoses. Rendering CTA images with inverted grayscale provides another format for image review that offers a different perspective on plaque composition.

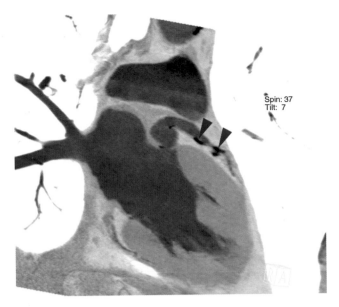

Figure 3.43 *Inverting the grayscale from Figure 41 highlights the LAD calcification* (arrowheads). Abbreviation: *LAD, left anterior descending artery.*

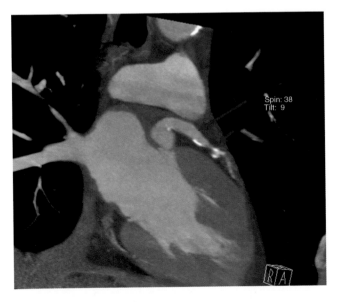

Figure 3.42 *CTA in an oblique plane similar to the right anterior oblique projection shows marked dilatation of the proximal LAD* (arrow) *with an abrupt change in vessel caliber* (short arrow). Abbreviation: *LAD, left anterior descending artery.*

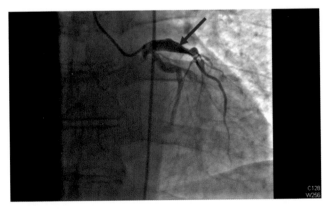

Figure 3.44 *Invasive coronary angiogram confirms the presence of LAD ectasia* (arrow).

CLINICAL CASE 17

A 58-year-old male with a history of repaired abdominal aortic aneurysm presented for further evaluation of a positive stress ECG.

CTA showed diffuse ectasia of the coronary arteries (**Figs. 3.45** and **3.46**), with left main measuring 7 mm, proximal LAD 9 mm, proximal left circumflex 6 mm, and proximal RCA 7 mm in diameter. Invasive angiography confirmed diffusely ectatic coronary arteries (**Fig. 3.47**).

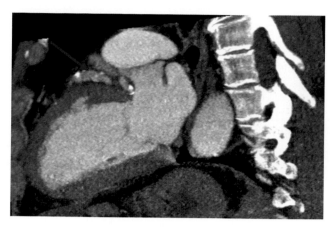

Figure 3.46 *Reformatted image in a vertical long axis plane shows the LAD ectasia* (arrow). *Note the presence of serial calcific plaque in this coronary artery.* Abbreviation: *LAD, left anterior descending artery.*

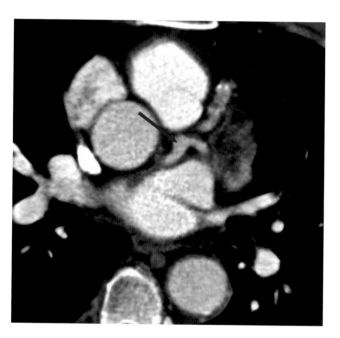

Figure 3.45 *Diffuse ectasia of the left mainstem* (arrow) *and proximal left anterior descending* (short arrow) *coronary arteries by CTA in an oblique axial plane.*

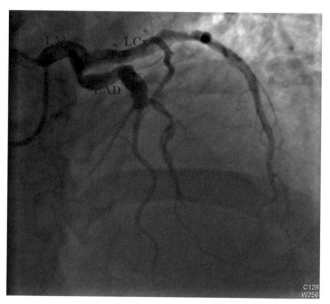

Figure 3.47 *Invasive coronary angiography confirms the presence of severe multivessel ectasia.* Abbreviations: *LM, left mainstem; LAD, left anterior descending artery; LCx, left circumflex coronary artery.*

ANEURYSM (KAWASAKI'S DISEASE)

CLINICAL CASE 18

A 15-year-old male with Kawasaki's disease in childhood presented for evaluation in adolescence. Given angiographic findings of coronary aneurysms during his childhood illness, he was referred for coronary CTA for follow-up assessment. CTA showed a 9 mm aneurysm in the proximal LAD (**Fig. 3.48**) and an 8 mm aneurysm in the proximal RCA (**Fig. 3.49**). The aneurysms appeared free of thrombus or atherosclerosis.

Role of CTA: Follow-up assessment of coronary artery aneurysms, deemed "giant" if greater than 10 mm in diameter, is imperative for young patients with a history of Kawasaki disease and coronary involvement. The long-term risks of rupture, thrombus formation, may be minimized with serial assessment that can be done noninvasively with CTA. These vessels may also develop atherosclerotic changes and stenosis, readily apparent by CTA.

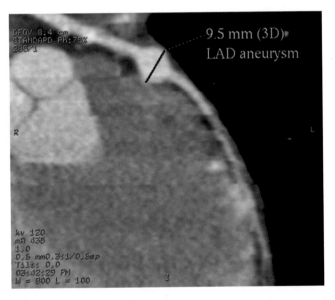

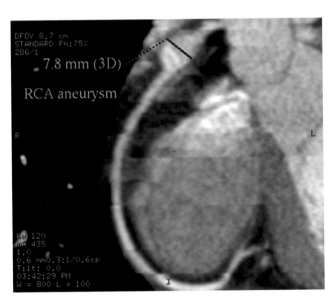

Figure 3.48 *Proximal left anterior descending coronary artery aneurysm in a patient with a history of Kawasaki's disease. Note the ability to measure the size of the coronary artery aneurysm noninvasively with CTA.*

Figure 3.49 *Reformatted CTA image of the right coronary artery in the same patient, demonstrating a 7.8 mm proximal RCA aneurysm.* Abbreviation: *RCA, right coronary artery.*

FISTULAS

CLINICAL CASE 19

A 58-year-old female with CAD and prior bypass surgery presented for evaluation of dyspnea. Invasive angiography showed patent LIMA to mid-LAD, SVG to RCA, and occluded SVG to OM. There was also suggestion of extracardiac communication of contrast during RCA injection (**Fig. 3.50**). She was referred for CTA for further definition.

CTA confirmed two of three grafts patent and also visualized a fistulous communication between the RCA and the right pulmonary artery (**Fig. 3.51**). CMR showed normal myocardial perfusion in all segments at rest and with vasodilator stress, and no significant net left-to-right shunt with Qp:Qs = 1:1.

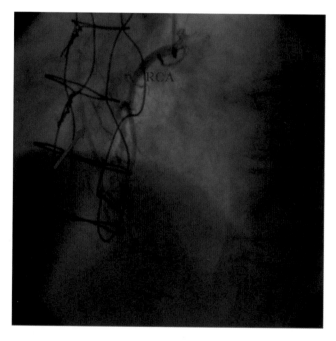

Figure 3.50 *Appearance of contrast in a vessel traveling away from the heart* (arrow) *with injection of contrast into the RCA.* Abbreviation: *RCA, right coronary artery.*

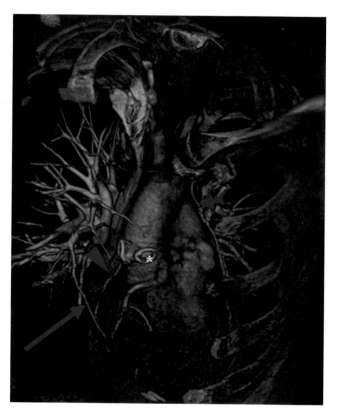

Figure 3.51 *Three-dimensional volume rendition of the CTA data illustrates the fistulous connection is between the RCA and a branch of the RPA* (arrow). *Also note the presence of a patent SVG to RCA* (arrowhead), *occluded SVG at the aortic anastomosis* (*), *and patent LIMA to LAD* (short arrow). Abbreviations: *LAD, left anterior descending artery; LIMA, left internal mammary artery; RCA, right coronary artery.*

CLINICAL CASE 20

A 63-year-old male who was seven years status-post orthotopic heart transplantation presented for annual evaluation. Physical examination revealed a right-sided S4 gallop.

CTA demonstrated a fistulous connection between the LAD and the right ventricle (RV) along the septum (**Fig. 3.52**), a typical site for endomyocardial biopsy sampling, which was confirmed with invasive angiography (**Fig. 3.53**).

Role of CTA: Volume rendering was able to demonstrate the relationship of the coronary vessel to the abnormal focal contrast enhancement in the RV cavity as well as the normal contrast-filled LV cavity. While this information could also be gleaned by review of the axial images, volume rendering that showed both the surface vessel and the cardiac chambers helped confirm the likely mechanism in this case, which was a coronary-to-RV fistula.

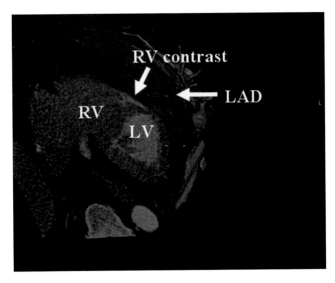

Figure 3.52 *CTA in a post-transplant patient shows localized contrast in the RV just below the left anterior descending coronary artery along the interventricular septum, consistent with coronary-to-RV fistula.* Abbreviations: *RV, right ventricle; LV, left ventricle.*

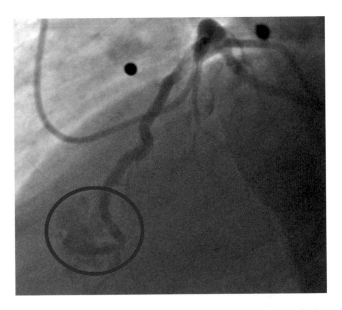

Figure 3.53 *Selective invasive angiography of the LAD shows a blush of contrast in the RV cavity during injection* (circle), *confirming the presence of a coronary-to-RV fistula.* Abbreviations: *RV, right ventricle; LAD, left anterior descending artery.*

BRIDGING

CLINICAL CASE 21

A 59-year-old obese male smoker with diabetes, hypertension, and obstructive sleep apnea presented for evaluation of worsening dyspnea and lower extremity edema. Nuclear stress testing was nondiagnostic due to attenuation artifact. Prior invasive coronary angiography had been unremarkable except for a short bridging segment of the LAD. In light of this history, he was referred for noninvasive CTA.

CTA redemonstrated that the mid-LAD took a short intramyocardial course (**Fig. 3.54**).

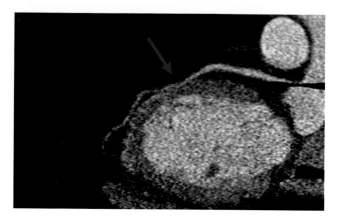

Figure 3.54 *CTA reformatted in an oblique sagittal plane demonstrates a short intramyocardial segment of the mid-left anterior descending coronary artery (arrow) that appeared most pronounced during systole. Note the relative graininess of the image due to obesity combined with ECG dose modulation that reduced the dose applied during systole. An alternative approach when bridging is suspected* a priori *is to not apply ECG dose modulation.* Abbreviation: *ECG, electrocardiogram.*

CORONARY SPASM

CLINICAL CASE 22

A 38-year-old female underwent CTA for evaluation of episodic chest pain not related to exertion. She had no risk factors for CAD, but did report a history of Raynaud's phenomenon. The coronary segments were free of atherosclerosis, though the proximal LAD had a beaded appearance, particularly when compared to the other coronary artery segments (**Fig. 3.55**). She proceeded to undergo invasive coronary cardiac catheterization; upon catheter engagement of the left main coronary ostium, the distal mainstem and proximal LAD underwent vasospasm with reproduction of her chest pain. Both the spasm and the symptoms resolved with intracoronary nitroglycerin.

Role of CTA: Notably, this patient had CTA examination completed without supplemental nitroglycerin administration. It is uncertain if this finding would have been feasible in the current era of nitroglycerin-enhanced coronary CTA.

(A)   (B)

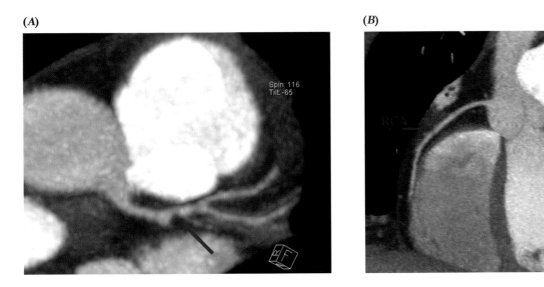

Figure 3.55 *Multiplanar reformatted CTA images demonstrate a beaded appearance of the proximal LAD (A, arrow) which may present as substrate for vessel spasm. In comparison, the remaining left and right coronary artery segments appear completely normal (B).*

CLINICAL PEARLS

- CTA can identify calcified, noncalcified, and mixed plaque in the coronary arteries.
- Nuclear stress testing may produce both false-positive and false-negative results; coronary CTA can make the correct diagnosis of the presence or absence of CAD.
- CTA may be limited in visualizing the lumen of coronary arteries with severe calcification; in such instances, functional assessment with modalities such as stress perfusion CMR provides complementary information on the hemodynamic significance of excessively calcified vessels.
- CTA may detect early coronary artery plaque in the absence of luminal obstruction, which may be missed with conventional invasive angiography or stress testing.
- Positive vessel wall remodeling also known as the Glagov phenomenon, which is associated with increased risk of plaque rupture, may be identified and quantified noninvasively with coronary CTA.
- CTA can readily delineate 3-D graft anatomy with volume rendering as well as graft patency with two-dimensional (2-D) image reconstruction.
- Prior to revascularization, suitable conduits such as the internal mammary arteries can be visualized with CTA.
- In patients who require repeat surgical revascularization, CTA can provide measurements of the distance from the chest well to the most anterior conduit such as a LIMA anastomosed to an LAD. This may help prevent iatrogenic injury to patent substernal conduits during repeat sternotomy.

- Some coronary artery stents can be assessed with CTA, particularly with the use of the appropriate reconstruction kernel along with cross-sectional and longitudinal 2-D reformatted images. Detection of in-stent restenosis, however, maybe limited in stents with a diameter <3.0mm due to partial volume effects and blooming artifacts.
- CTA provides a mechanism of detecting ostial coronary artery or bypass graft disease noninvasively. This may be preferred to invasive angiography with its attendant risk of catheter-induced ischemia due to occlusion of a vessel with high-grade ostial disease.
- Both coronary artery aneurysms and ectasia can be appreciated with CTA, allowing noninvasive serial assessment that may be particularly useful in patients with disorders such as Kawasaki's disease.
- Evaluation of the patient after orthotopic heart transplantation, who has undergone endomyocardial biopsy, should include assessment not only for CAD but also for unusual complications such as coronary-to-RV fistulas.
- Prior knowledge of a bridging coronary artery segment might warrant CTA acquisition without ECG dose modulation applied, insuring sufficient image quality during systolic phases when compression of the bridging segment occurs.
- The irregular coronary lumen in the absence of atherosclerotic disease should raise the suspicion of a vasospastic segment, particularly within the appropriate clinical context.

Chapter 4   Coronary anomalies

Anomalies of coronary artery anatomy, typically categorized on the basis of location of origin from the aorta and proximal course, are thought to be present in approximately 1% of the general population. The first manifestation of certain forms of coronary artery anomaly may be sudden death. Coronary anomalies are thought to represent 19% of all cases of sudden death in young (age <35 years) athletes. Therefore, correct identification and precise definition of the anatomic course of the coronary arteries are of great importance, particularly when evaluating symptomatic athletes. Precise definitions of sudden death mechanisms due to coronary anomaly remain elusive, though it is thought that extrinsic compression interrupts coronary flow in anomalies that take an interarterial course between the aorta and the right ventricular outflow tract. Patients with interarterial segments may undergo intervention such as bypass surgery to redirect the blood flow to the myocardium, while other anomalies not associated with sudden death may warrant observation alone.

The imaging protocol for coronary anomalies is no different than that for imaging normal coronary arteries. However, in the case of computed tomography (CT) imaging in children, certain modifications of the normal protocol are undertaken. First, we limit the volume of coverage to the heart, whenever possible; this is identified from the initial tomogram. Scanning more than a few centimeters above the aortic root or below the base of the heart is unnecessary for coronary imaging and increases the overall radiation dose of the study. Lower kVp and mAs (tube voltage and current settings, respectively) are selected for the scan acquisition parameters; this does not significantly affect image quality in children who tend to have a lower body mass than adults with less soft tissue attenuation of the incident X rays. Additionally, the use of lead aprons placed over the lower abdomen and thyroid shields placed on the patient during scanning, similar to those worn in the heart catheterization laboratory, limit exposure to susceptible organs.

CLINICAL CASE 1

A 57-year-old male presented for evaluation of chest pain. Invasive angiography demonstrated that the left coronary artery (LCA) originated from the right sinus of Valsalva, though the proximal course could not be determined with certainty. Given the risk of sudden cardiac death with anomalous coronary arteries that take an interarterial course between the great vessels, the patient was referred for CT angiography (CTA) to define this three-dimensional anatomy.

CTA showed a single coronary artery ostium arising from the right sinus of Valsalva. The LCA was shown to take an interarterial course between aorta and right ventricular outflow tract by both multiplanar reformatted imaging (**Fig. 4.1**) and volume rendering (**Fig. 4.2**). The right coronary artery (RCA) was without significant obstructive disease. Based on these findings, he underwent two-vessel surgical revascularization consisting of an internal mammary artery conduit to the left anterior descending coronary artery (LAD) and saphenous vein graft to an obtuse marginal branch of the left circumflex coronary artery (LCx), thus completely bypassing the anomalous LCA origin.

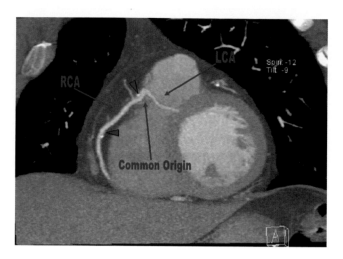

Figure 4.1 *Anomalous origin of the LCA from the right sinus of Valsalva. Note the nonobstructive plaque in the RCA* (arrowheads). Abbreviations: *LCA, left coronary artery; RCA, right coronary artery.*

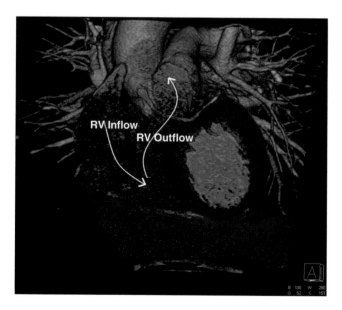

Figure 4.2 *Interarterial course of the LCA* (arrowhead) *shown beneath the right ventricular outflow tract, which has been cut away in this volume-rendered image.* Abbreviation: *LCA, left coronary artery.*

CLINICAL CASE 2

An obese 55-year-old female with hypertension, hyperlipidemia, and family history of premature atherosclerosis presented for evaluation of chest pain.

CTA showed an anomalous left main coronary artery originating from the right sinus of Valsalva, taking an interarterial course between the right ventricular outflow tract and aorta (**Figs. 4.3** and **4.4**). The RCA had a normal course. On the basis of these findings, she was referred for bypass surgery of the LCA.

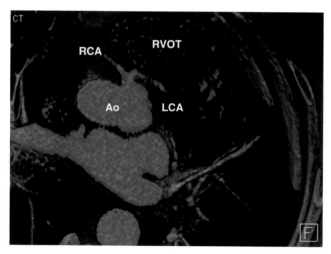

Figure 4.3 *An anomalous LCA takes an interarterial course between the aorta* (Ao) *and the right ventricular outflow tract. The single coronary ostium is demonstrated as the RCA emanates from the same location.* Abbreviations: *LCA, left coronary artery; RCA, right coronary artery.*

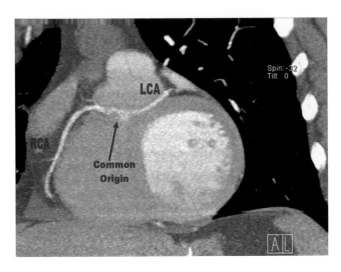

Figure 4.4 *MPR in a left anterior oblique projection demonstrates the common origin of the coronary arteries from the right sinus of Valsalva.* Abbreviation: *MPR, multiplanar reformatted image.*

CLINICAL CASE 3

A 23-year-old female with congenital heart disease status post right ventricle (RV) to main pulmonary artery conduit underwent CTA for follow-up. This demonstrated the proximal RCA coursing between the native right ventricular outflow tract and the RV–conduit (**Fig. 4.5**).

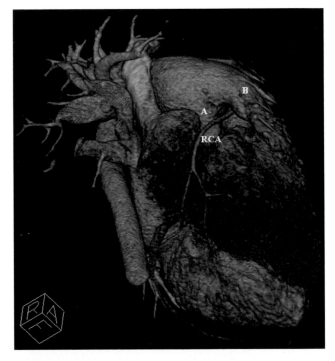

Figure 4.5 *An RCA in a patient with repaired congenital heart disease travels anterior to the native right ventricular outflow tract (A) but beneath the RV–PA conduit (B).* Abbreviations: *RV, right ventricle; PA, pulmonary artery; RCA, right coronary artery.*

CLINICAL CASE 4

A 73-year-old male with multiple risk factors for coronary artery disease presented for coronary CTA. This showed an anomalous origin of the left main coronary artery from the right aortic sinus, taking an interarterial course between the aorta and the RV outflow tract (**Fig. 4.6**).

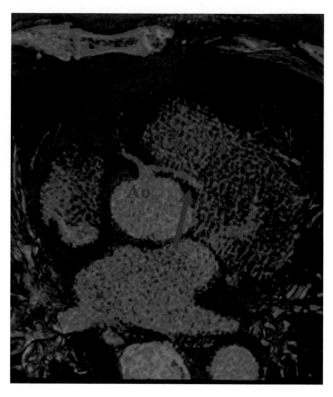

Figure 4.6   *An anomalous left main coronary artery* (arrow) *arising from a single coronary ostium off of the right sinus of Valsalva with an interarterial course.* Abbreviations: *Ao, aorta; RVOT, right ventricular outflow tract.*

ANOMALOUS ORIGIN AND OTHER PROXIMAL COURSE VARIANTS

CLINICAL CASE 5

A 69-year-old male smoker with hypertension presented for the evaluation of coronary artery disease. CTA showed that the ostium of the RCA was superior and leftward from its usual position off of the right sinus of Valsalva (**Fig. 4.7**). No obstructive disease was visualized.

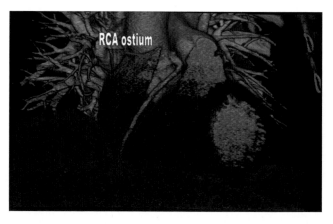

Figure 4.7   *Volume rendering of the CTA data demonstrates a superior, leftward origin of the RCA.* Abbreviation: *RCA, right coronary artery.*

CLINICAL CASE 6

A 24-year-old male with D-type transposition of the great arteries status post Mustard repair presented for routine follow-up evaluation. CTA (**Fig. 4.8**) showed the both the LAD and the RCA arising from the left sinus of Valsalva from distinct coronary ostia, but with no interarterial segments.

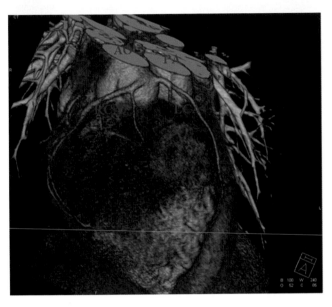

Figure 4.8 *Volume rendering shows distinct origins of the dominant right and nondominant left coronary arteries (RCA, LCA) from the left sinus of Valsalva. Note the relatively larger right coronary artery supplying a systemic right ventricle in this patient with repaired D-type transposition of the great arteries. Abbreviations: Ao, aorta; PA, main pulmonary artery.*

CLINICAL CASE 7

A 24-year-old female with congenital pulmonic stenosis status post childhood repair presented for routine follow-up with CTA. This demonstrated a common right coronary/LAD ostium arising from the right sinus of Valsalva, with the LAD coursing anterior to the right ventricular outflow tract (**Fig. 4.9**). The left circumflex originated distinctly from the left sinus of Valsalva (**Fig. 4.10**). No atherosclerosis was visualized in the coronary arteries.

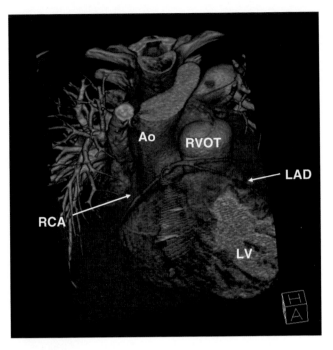

Figure 4.9 *Anomalous LAD from a common ostium with the RCA. Abbreviations: RCA, right coronary artery; LAD, left anterior descending coronary artery.*

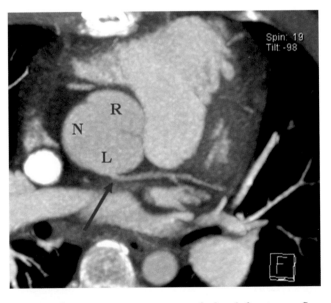

Figure 4.10 *Distinct ostium of the left circumflex* (arrow) *in the same patient from the left sinus of Valsalva. The sinuses are labeled left (L), right (R), and noncoronary (N).*

CLINICAL CASE 8

A 52-year-old male presented for evaluation of substernal chest pain. Coronary CTA showed separate ostia of the left circumflex and LAD from the left aortic sinus of Valsalva. There is also severe narrowing in the proximal segment of the left circumflex artery (**Fig. 4.11**), caused by a noncalcified atherosclerotic plaque.

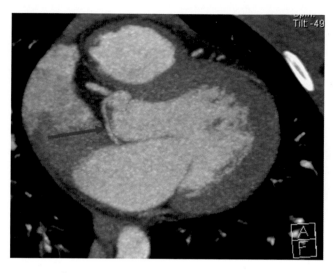

Figure 4.12 *Axial maximum intensity projection image demonstrates the anomalous left circumflex coronary artery arising from the right sinus of Valsalva (arrow).*

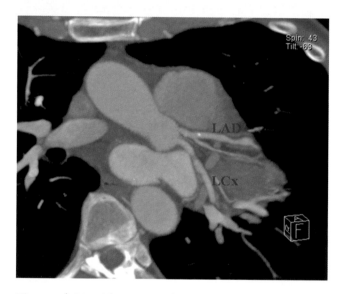

Figure 4.11 *The circumflex (LCx) and left anterior descending coronary arteries (LAD) arise from distinct ostia directly from the left sinus of Valsalva without a left mainstem segment.*

CLINICAL CASE 9

An 18-year-old male with congenitally bicuspid aortic valve was referred for CTA prior to surgery. This demonstrated an anomalous left circumflex arising from the right sinus of Valsalva and traveling posterior to the aorta (**Figs. 4.12** and **4.13**).

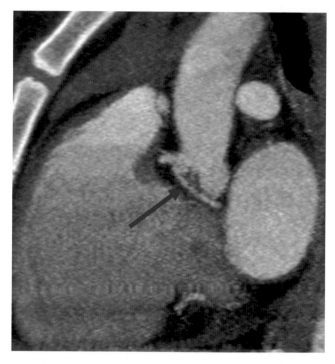

Figure 4.13 *Sagittal multiplanar reformatted image shows the anomalous circumflex coronary artery arising from the right sinus of Valsalva (arrow).*

CLINICAL CASE 10

A 68-year-old male with a known coronary artery anomaly, managed medically, was referred for coronary CTA to define the origins and proximal courses of the coronary arteries. Invasive angiography showed a single coronary artery arising from the right cusp (**Fig. 4.14**), and no coronary artery was seen with injection in the left coronary cusp (**Fig. 4.15**). CTA was subsequently performed, documenting an interarterial course of the left main coronary artery (**Figs. 4.16** and **4.17**). The RCA was seen in its appropriate location (**Fig. 4.18**).

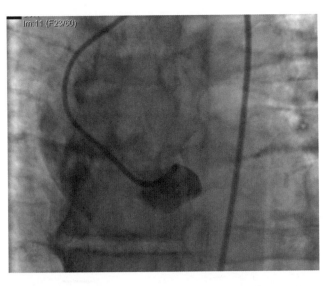

Figure 4.15 *Selective injection with a left coronary catheter shows no coronary artery arising from the left sinus of Valsalva (*).*

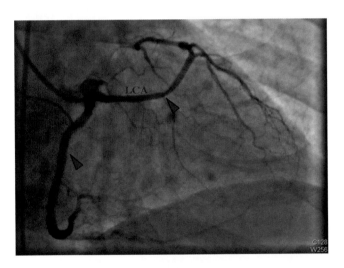

Figure 4.14 *Selective invasive coronary angiography using a right coronary catheter in the right sinus of Valsalva opacifies the entire coronary artery tree. Mild luminal irregularities are suggestive of atherosclerotic plaque* (arrowheads), *which is better demonstrated with CTA. Abbreviations: RCA, right coronary artery; LCA, left coronary artery.*

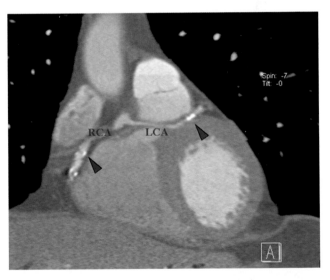

Figure 4.16 *MPR demonstrating the anomalous single coronary ostium. Note the atherosclerotic plaque that is more apparent than that seen by catheter-based lumenography alone* (arrowheads). *Abbreviations: LCA, left coronary artery; RCA, right coronary artery; MPR, multiplanar reformatted image.*

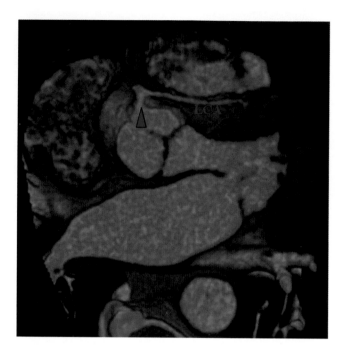

Figure 4.17 *Volume rendering of the common coronary ostium* (arrowhead) *demonstrating both the anomalous origin and the interarterial course of the left coronary artery.*

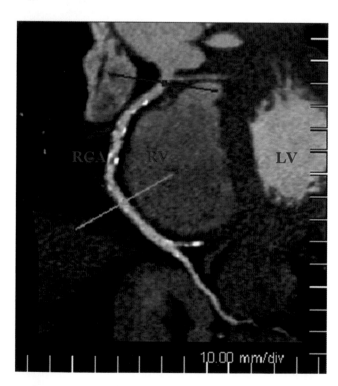

Figure 4.18 *The RCA is a large, dominant vessel seen with diffuse atherosclerotic plaque along its entire length.* Abbreviations: *RCA, right coronary artery; RV, right ventricle; LV, left ventricle.*

CLINICAL CASE 11

A 36-year-old male with aortic coarctation and bicuspid aortic valve presented for follow-up evaluation of the aorta and coronary arteries. CTA showed the anomalous origin of the left circumflex arising from a distinct right sinus of Valsalva ostium and coursing posterior to the aorta (**Fig. 4.19**). Similar anatomy from a different case is shown in **Fig. 4.22**.

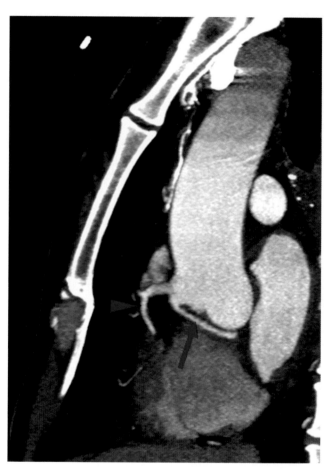

Figure 4.19 *Anomalous and distinct ostium of the left circumflex coronary artery* (arrow) *from the anterior right sinus of Valsalva. Note the adjacent right coronary artery* (arrowhead) *is also seen in this projection.*

CLINICAL CASE 12

A 26-year-old male with repaired D-transposition of the great arteries underwent CTA for follow-up.

This demonstrated the relationship of the great vessels to each other, as well as the orientation of the aortic sinuses with the right and left coronary artery ostia (**Figs. 4.20** and **4.21**).

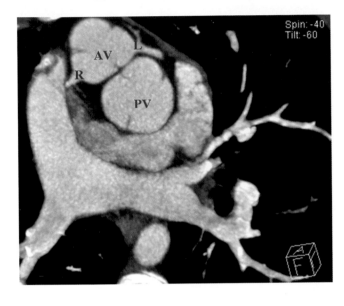

Figure 4.20 *Oblique axial MPR image demonstrates that in this patient with repaired D-transposition of the great arteries, the AV is anterior and slightly rightward to the PV with altered configuration of the aortic sinuses of Valsalva resulting in a unique anatomy of the right (R) and left (L) coronary arteries. Abbreviations: AV, aortic valve; MPR, multiplanar reformatted image; PV, pulmonic valve.*

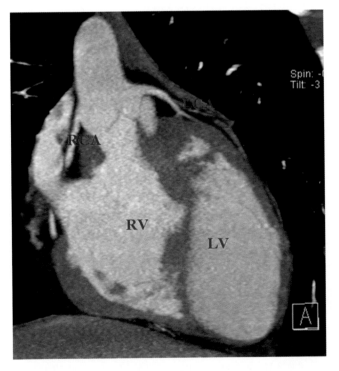

Figure 4.21 *Coronal reformatted CTA image demonstrates the proximal course of both the left and the right coronary arteries (LCA, RCA) from the aorta in a patient with repaired D-transposition of the great arteries. Note the hypertrophied systemic RV compared to the thin-walled pulmonary LV. Abbreviations: RV, right ventricle; LV, left ventricle.*

(A)

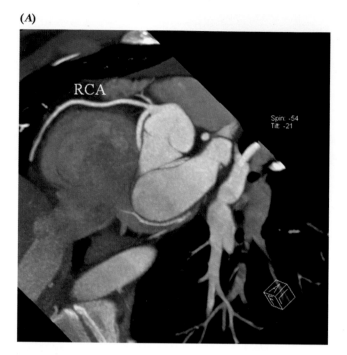

(B)

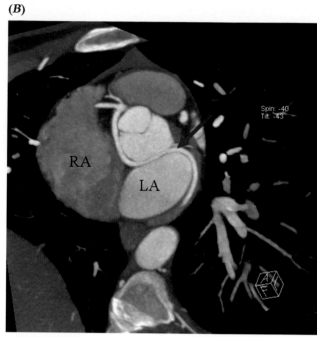

Figure 4.22   *Maximum intensity projection CT images in different oblique planes demonstrate another example of anomalous origin of the left circumflex artery from the right sinus of Valsalva (similar to Fig. 19). The circumflex artery* (arrow) *travels posterior to the aorta around the LA.* Abbreviations: *RCA, right coronary artery; RA, right atrium; LA, left atrium; CT, computed tomography.*

CLINICAL PEARLS

- CTA readily demonstrates both the origin and the course of the coronary arteries, either or both of which may be anomalous.
- CTA can identify anomalous coronary artery variations that are associated with sudden cardiac death, such as those that take an inter-arterial course between the great vessels. Referral for surgical revascularization may be indicated in such cases.
- Various forms of congenital heart disease are associated with coronary artery anomalies, which can be easily delineated using coronary CTA. Recognition of these anomalies is important for patients who may require repeat surgery to avoid iatrogenic injury to the coronary arteries.
- Localization of anomalous coronary artery ostia is helpful in patients who require invasive angiography, because this may require selection

- of different diagnostic and guide catheters for selective injection and intervention.
- Invasive angiography is limited in defining the three-dimensional anatomy of anomalous coronary arteries; in such cases, CTA can provide definitive visualization of the coronary arteries and their relationship to the great vessels.
- In many patients, particularly of younger age, "unroofing" surgical procedures are preferred to bypass surgery. By providing complete three-dimensional anatomy of the coronary artery origin, course, and its relationship to the aorta, CT easily identifies patients that are candidates for this type of surgical repair.
- Anomalous coronary arteries may also develop atherosclerotic plaque that can be visualized with CTA.

Chapter 5   **Artifacts**

A computed tomography (CT) image artifact is defined as "any discrepancy between the reconstructed CT numbers in the image and the true attenuation coefficients of the object" (1).

Potential sources of artifact include the patient (e.g., breathing or other motion), the imaging technique (e.g., improper calibration), and the imaging equipment (e.g., ring artifact due to faulty detectors). Artifacts can also be classified on the basis of their appearance: streaks, shadings, or rings. Streaks, straight lines of artifact across the image, may result from metal, beam hardening, patient motion, or improper table speed (pitch) selection. Shading, which may occur near objects of high densities or as a result of scattered radiation, may result in a darker intensity than would actually be produced by the object.

COMMON ARTIFACTS

PATIENT MOTION

Patient motion artifacts can be voluntary or involuntary (**Figs. 5.1** and **5.2**). Swallowing or respiration can affect image quality but can be controlled by the patient; prescan instructions are critical to educate the patient and minimize voluntary motion–induced artifact. Artifacts due to involuntary motion such as the beating of the heart or irregularities due to arrhythmias (**Fig. 5.5**) may occur with cardiac CT imaging. Both motion artifacts will appear as streaks or "stair steps" that result from data inconsistencies not recognized by the reconstruction algorithm. Decreasing scan time and limiting image reconstruction to phases of the cardiac cycle with minimal motion (e.g., end-diastole) can help minimize cardiac motion–induced artifacts.

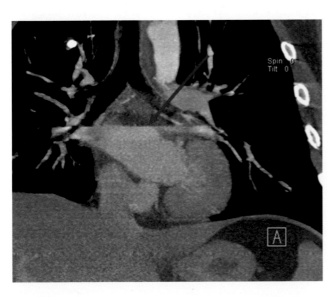

Figure 5.1 *Marked artifact due to motion appears as a horizontal line at the location of the gantry when motion occurred.*

(A)

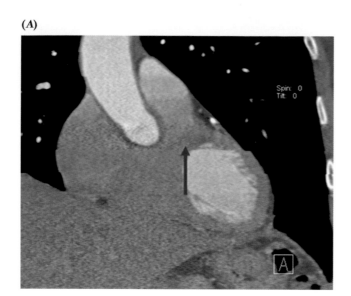

(B)

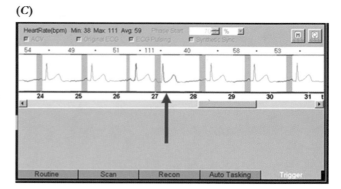

(C)

Figure 5.2 *(A) A horizontal line in the coronal reformatted plane that represents a premature atrial beat that occurred during the acquisition. (B) A horizontal line in the sagittal reformatted plane that represents a premature atrial beat that occurred during the acquisition. Note similar shifts in the chest wall. (C) The recorded electrocardiographic signal captures the premature atrial complex that occurred during the acquisition.*

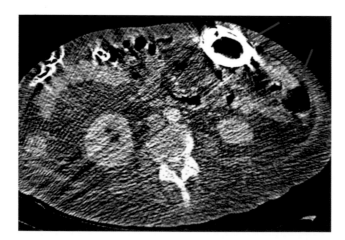

Figure 5.3 *Severe streak artifacts in a patient with a left ventricular assist device. The inflow and outflow cannulae are seen in cross-section (arrows) (also see Chapter 6).*

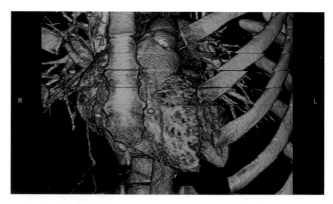

Figure 5.4 *Step artifact is quite prominent in this patient who had significant difficulty with even brief breathholding.*

(A)

(B)

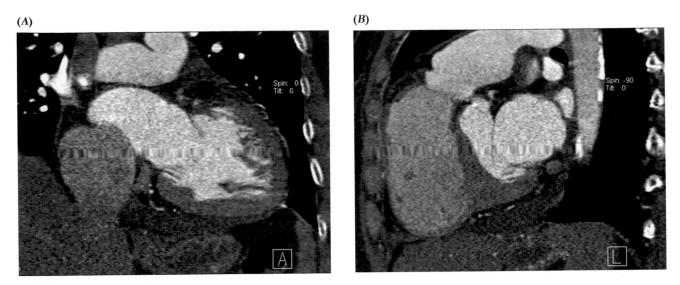

Figure 5.5 *Illustration of band-like artifact in a patient with an irregular heart rate; removal of data in an attempt to minimize artifact due to an ectopic beat results in incomplete data, causing the band seen across the heart in the anterior and sagittal reformatted images.*

METAL ARTIFACTS

Metal such as cardiac pacemakers, surgical clips, and electrodes can generate streak artifacts. The metal object absorbs the radiation, resulting in incomplete projection profiles. External metal objects should be removed from the field of view whenever possible. Pacemaker and defibrillator leads in the right heart can interfere significantly with visualization of the right coronary artery (**Fig. 5.6**). Other intracardiac devices such as coronary stents may obscure the segment of interest, though use of sharper reconstruction kernels (Chapter 1) may help improve intraluminal visualization in stented segments.

(A)

(B)

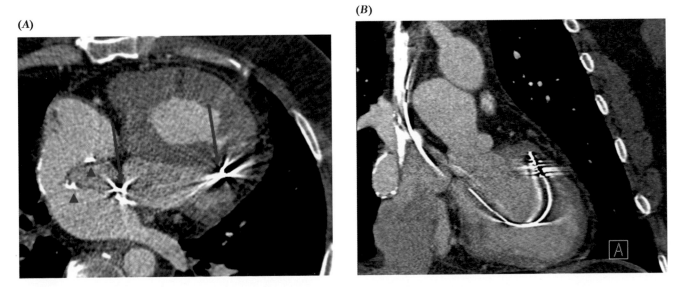

Figure 5.6 *Artifact due to pacemaker leads (arrows). Also note calcification within the pulmonary venous baffle in this patient with d-transposition of the great arteries (arrowheads).*

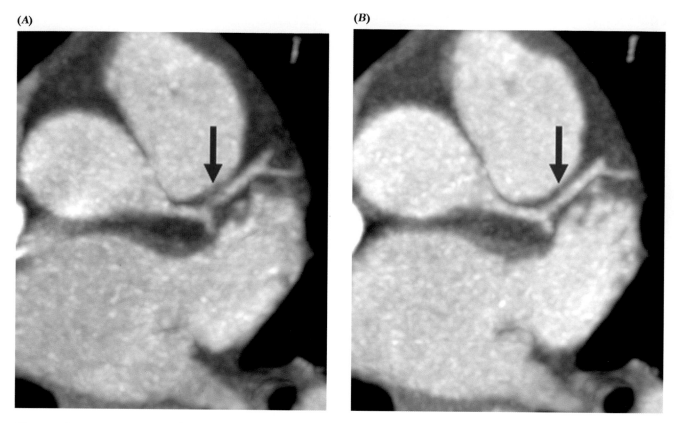

Figure 5.7 *Appearance of a possible stenosis in the proximal LAD with image review at 75% of the R–R interval (**A**). With selection of a different cardiac phase for reformatting (60%, **B**), this coronary segment appears normal consistent with cardiac motion–induced artifact. This problem can also be corrected by reconstructing the images after editing (deleting) data collected during the premature beat.* Abbreviation: *LAD, left anterior descending artery.*

BEAM-HARDENING ARTIFACTS

Beam hardening refers to the increase in the mean energy of the x-ray beam as it passes through the patient. As the object size increases, the mean energy shifts because lower energy photons are preferentially absorbed. This causes the CT numbers of certain structures to change, creating artifacts. Beam hardening can also occur when the radiation beams have different path lengths. The path is longer in the center of the object and shorter at the periphery, affecting the resultant CT numbers. These changes appear as broad dark bands or streaks. Software advances have minimized artifacts from structures like the skull; in the heart, beam hardening may occur due to high iodine contrast concentration or calcification.

PARTIAL VOLUME ARTIFACTS

CT numbers are based on attenuation coefficients for a voxel of tissue. If the voxel contains only one tissue type, there is not a problem. If the voxel contains more than one tissue type, then the CT number will be based on the average of the different tissues. A dense calcified plaque or the walls of a stent may appear to have a larger size due to partial volume effects, creating an exaggerated narrowing of the coronary artery. This problem is magnified if in addition there is a motion artifact. Partial volume artifacts are reduced with slice scans and computer algorithms.

NOISE-INDUCED ARTIFACTS

The number of photons that strike the detectors directly influences the noise. More photons mean less noise and better image quality. Increased noise will lead to streak artifacts or an excessively grainy appearance of the resultant images.

Increased noise can be a result of soft tissue attenuation as with obesity (**Fig. 5.8**), improper selection of technique factors (kVp, mA), and incorrect scan speed (pitch). Optimization of all of these factors can reduce noise-induced artifacts.

(B)

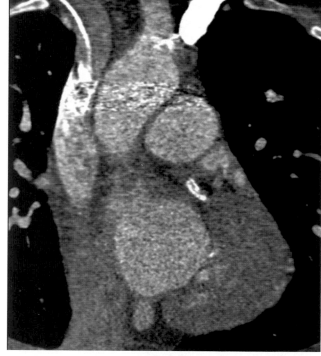

(A)

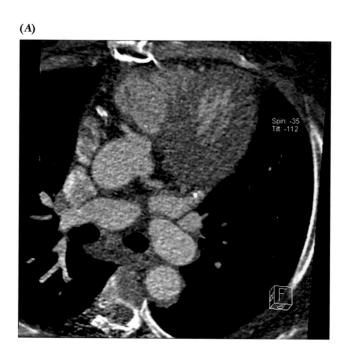

(C)

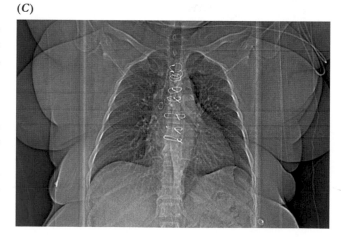

Figure 5.8   *Illustration of noise caused by obesity. The penetration of the X rays is modulated by the excess body tissue, causing the grainy appearance of the entire image including the coronaries (axial and coronal reformatted computed tomography images, **A** and **B**, respectively). The presence of a tremendous amount of soft tissue in this patient can be appreciated upon inspection of the topogram (**C**). Image manipulation cannot mitigate the grainy quality of the image. Extra contrast can be delivered for enhanced opacification or the coronaries or other vascular structures in this situation; this will ease interpretation of the images despite overall limitations in signal intensity.*

OTHER ARTIFACTS

Selection of the appropriate cardiac phase for reconstruction of images helps insure good image quality; artifact may result from both cardiac motion, particularly during systolic phases, and increased noise, if using dose-modulation. In the latter case, radiation dose is reduced to 20% of the full dose during the systolic phases; reconstruction of images during the systolic phases may, therefore, result in stairstep-like artifact and increased noise due to decreased signal-to-noise ratio in the setting of reduced radiation dose (**Fig. 5.9**). Poor timing of contrast delivery results in poor image quality and limited interpretation of the structures of interest. **Figure 5.10** illustrates acquisition obtained too early for optimal coronary opacification, with significant contrast remaining in the right heart. Appropriate timing of acquisition insures that contrast opacifies the structures of interest.

(B)

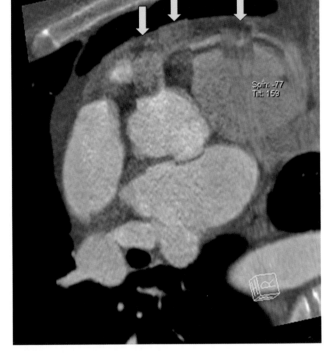

(A)

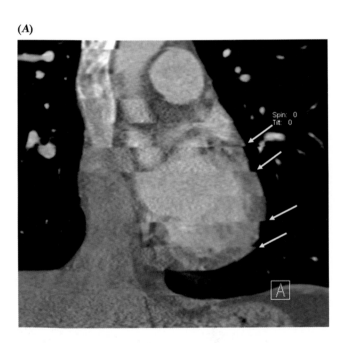

Figure 5.9   (Continued)

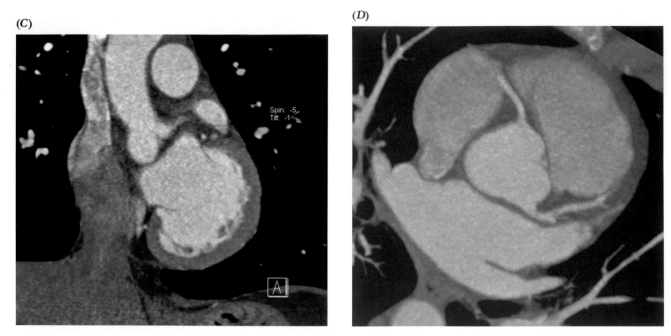

Figure 5.9 (Continued) *Cardiac phase artifact. (**A**) and (**B**) are different reformatted planes of the same systolic phase (35% of the R–R interval). Note the prominent stairstep-type appearance throughout the cardiac structures imaged in these planes. Below, in (**C**) and (**D**), the same planes are illustrated, only with the choice of a diastolic phase (70% in this case) of the cardiac cycle for reconstruction. The stairstep artifact is almost completely eliminated, highlighting the importance of choosing the correct phase from which to reconstruct the acquired image data. This is an interactive process; different segments of the coronary tree may be optimally viewed at different phases, warranting review of multiple phases of thin section data at sites of potential lesions. Also note less graininess of the images reconstructed at 70% of the R–R interval due to full radiation dose application compared to ECG dose modulation, resulting in 20% of the full dose being applied at the 35% phase.* Abbreviation: *ECG, electrocardiogram.*

(A) (B)

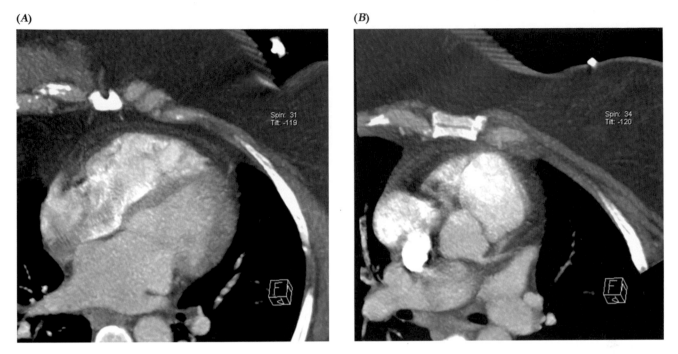

Figure 5.10 *Artifact due to inappropriate timing of contrast delivery. The views selected [(A) horizontal long axis and (B) oblique axial plane at the level of the pulmonary artery and aortic valve] reveal that this inappropriately early acquisition resulted in images with contrast opacifying the right heart and the pulmonary structures with poor opacification of the aortic root, coronary arteries, and left heart. Furthermore, high concentration of residual iodinated contrast in the superior vena cava (B) produces significant streak artifact.*

REFERENCE

1. Hsieh J. Image artifacts, causes and correction. In: Goldman LV, Fowlkes JB, eds. *Medical CT and Ultrasound: Current Technology and Applications*, 1995.

Chapter 6   **The left ventricle**

Imaging the left ventricle (LV) with gated cardiac computed tomography imaging is largely a matter of timing the contrast delivery. Optimal opacification of the LV cavity can be achieved by first performing a test bolus utilizing 10 to 20 cc of contrast and interactively determining the peak signal intensity of the contrast within the LV. Often, we will choose a time point that allows for good opacification of the LV as well as adequate opacification of the aortic root and coronary arteries for simultaneous coronary anatomy assessment. This time delay from the contrast injection time to the beginning of scan time is used during subsequent delivery of an 80 to 100 cc contrast bolus during volumetric (helical) image acquisition. Regular heart rate during both timing bolus and helical scans is key to (*i*) appropriate timing delay selection and (*ii*) images of LV myocardium that are free of cardiac motion artifact. Arrhythmias or ectopic beats can result in erratic multiphase cine images wherein the myocardial position at one phase of the cardiac cycle abruptly transitions to a nonadjacent phase location. This loss of temporal uniformity results in erroneous measurement of LV volumes and thickening,

underscoring again the importance of obtaining a regular, stable heart rhythm prior to scanning.

Electrocardiogram (ECG) dose modulation reduces the radiation dose to typically 20% of maximum dose during systolic phases of the cardiac cycle, reducing radiation exposure to the patient and maximizing energy transmission during diastole when coronary image reconstruction is preferred due to minimized vessel motion. This reduces signal-to-noise ratio for images reconstructed during the systolic phases, resulting in increased graininess of these phases of the cardiac cycle (see Chapter 5, Artifacts). This loss of image quality is rarely severe enough to render dynamic LV imaging uninterpretable; for example, there is still usually sufficient contrast at the endocardial border to measure systolic volumes with either border detection or signal intensity segmentation algorithms. For cases where high-resolution LV imaging throughout the cardiac cycle is needed, such as imaging of an intramyocardial bridging segment of a coronary artery, ECG dose modulation should be turned off, assuming that the need for increased image quality warrants the resulting increase in radiation dose.

NORMAL

CLINICAL CASE 1

A 56-year-old female with hypertension and family history of premature coronary artery disease (CAD) presented for evaluation of episodic, fleeting chest discomfort not reliably precipitated by exertion. Stress testing was borderline abnormal

and the patient was referred for a coronary CT angiography (CTA).

This showed normal left ventricular size and systolic function (**Fig. 6.1**), LV ejection fraction (EF) 60%, along with isolated plaque disease in the coronary arteries.

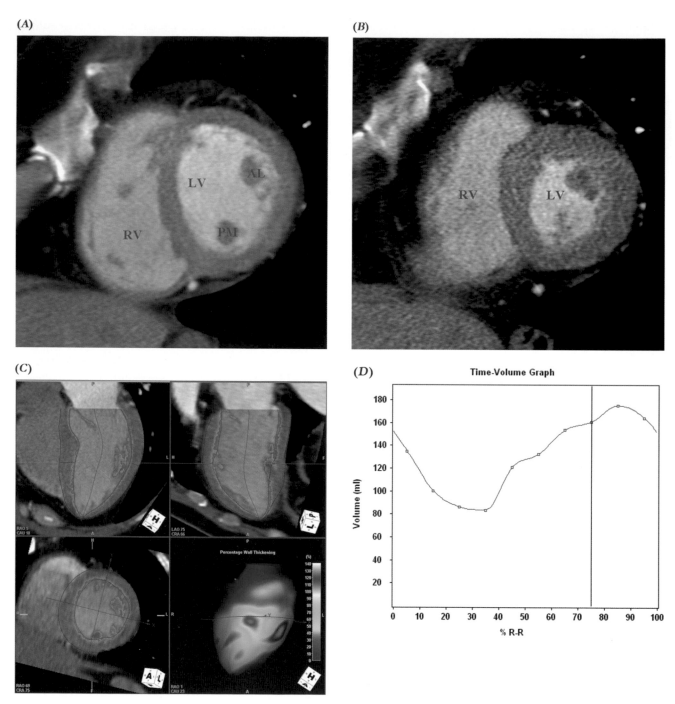

Figure 6.1   *End-diastolic (**A**) and end-systolic (**B**) maximum intensity projection images reformatted in the short-axis plane. Notice the difference between diastole (in which the papillary muscles are visible) and systole (in which the papillary muscles are bunched, LV myocardium is thickened, and the LV cavity is smaller). All segments of the myocardium are thickened at end-systole compared to end-diastole, indicating normal LV systolic function. There is mildly reduced signal-to-noise in the systolic image due to application of ECG dose modulation during the acquisition. This reduction in radiation dose exposure to the patient does not preclude delineation of the endocardial surface of the LV relative to the myocardium, resulting in adequate contrast at this interface for border detection and ejection fraction computation (**C**). (**D**) Time-volume curve, where time is expressed as a percentage of the R-R interval.* Abbreviations: *LV, left ventricle; RV, right ventricle; AL, anterolateral papillary muscle; PM, posteromedial papillary muscle; ECG, electrocardiogram.*

CLINICAL CASE 2

A 63-year-old female with asthma and prior aortic valve placement presented for evaluation of progressive dyspnea on exertion. Exercise stress testing was terminated at three minutes of the Bruce protocol due to fatigue and wheezing, which also precluded vasodilator stress, resulting in an inadequate assessment of myocardial ischemia. To assess for CAD as the etiology of her dyspnea, she was referred for coronary CTA. This provided suitable images for both coronary artery and left ventricular assessment, demonstrating normal coronary arteries and normal left ventricular size and systolic function (**Fig. 6.2**).

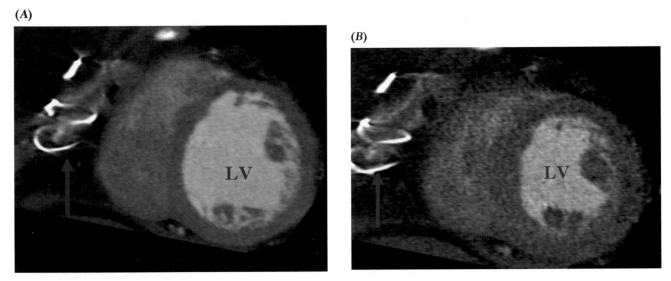

Figure 6.2 *End-diastolic (**A**) and end-systolic (**B**) images in a patient with sternal wires (arrows) who was unable to undergo adequate stress nuclear imaging show normal systolic function of the LV. As in Figure 1, ECG dose modulation results in slightly increased graininess of the systolic frame, though endocardium–myocardium contrast remains high. Abbreviations: LV, left ventricle; ECG, electrocardiogram.*

ABNORMAL LV FUNCTION

CLINICAL CASE 3

A 77-year-old male with hypertension, chronic obstructive pulmonary disease, hyperlipidemia, and prior coronary artery bypass surgery presented for evaluation of progressive fatigue. Given poor functional capacity and nondiagnostic stress testing in the past, as well as poor acoustic windows with echocardiography (**Figs. 6.3** and **6.4**), he was referred for coronary CTA to determine graft patency and LV function.

While severe calcification precluded visualization of the native coronary arteries, bypass grafts to all three coronary territories were shown to be patent:

left internal mammary artery to mid–left anterior descending artery, sequential saphenous vein graft (SVG) to obtuse marginal1, and SVG to distal right coronary artery. Analysis of multiphase reformatted images demonstrated LV dilatation (LVEDVI 89 mL/m², LVESVI 72 mL/m²) with moderately severe systolic dysfunction, (LV EF 19%), along with a myocardial perfusion abnormality suggestive of scar (**Fig. 6.5**). Cardiac magnetic resonance (CMR) with delayed post–gadolinium imaging confirmed moderately severe LV dilatation and systolic dysfunction (LVEDVI 92 mL/m², LVESVI 75 mL/m², LV EF 21%) and nontransmural scar involving the inferior and lateral walls (**Fig. 6.6**).

(A)

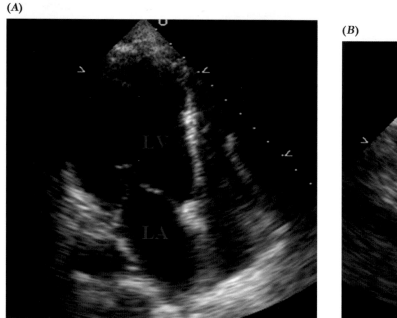

(B)

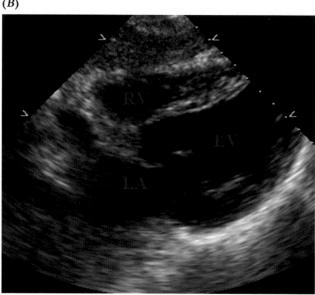

Figure 6.3 *Echocardiography images of fair quality from parasternal* (**A**) *and apical windows* (**B**). *Note the difficulty in visualizing the apex in this patient.* Abbreviations: *RV, right ventricle; LV, left ventricle; LA, left atrium.*

(A)

(B)

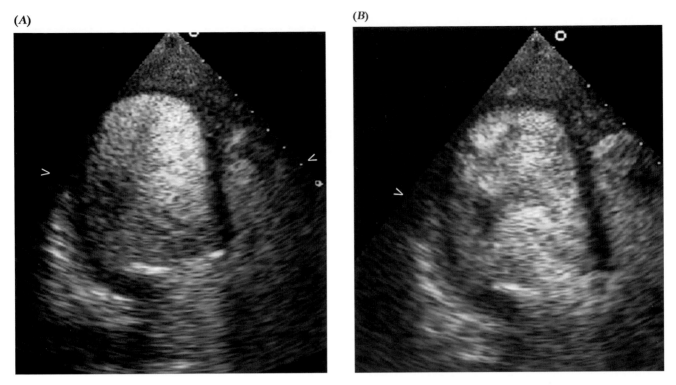

Figure 6.4 *Addition of a transpulmonic contrast agent helps with visualization of the LV apex noted both in diastole (**A**) and in systole (**B**).* Abbreviation: *LV, left ventricle.*

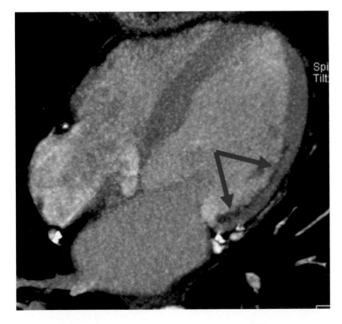

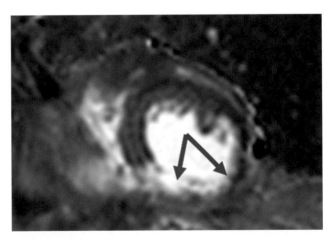

Figure 6.6 *Cardiac magnetic resonance delayed post–gadolinium image confirms the presence of nontransmural scar along the lateral wall* (arrow).

Figure 6.5 *CT angiography image reformatted in the HLA plane demonstrates a nontransmural perfusion defect (darker subendocardial region) along the antero-lateral wall* (arrows). Abbreviation: *HLA, horizontal long axis.*

A 59-year-old male with CAD status-post bypass surgery and implantable cardiac defibrillator placement presented for evaluation of chest tightness.

Nuclear stress testing demonstrated moderately reduced left ventricular systolic function with LV EF of 27% and no evidence of ischemia (**Fig. 6.7**). Coronary CTA showed left ventricular segmental dysfunction (**Fig. 6.8**) and dilatation that was quantified as follows: LVEDV 317 mL, LVESV 250 mL, and LV EF 21%. Four of four grafts were patent.

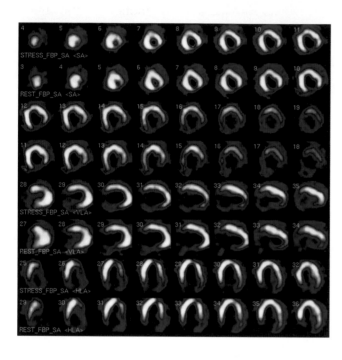

Figure 6.7 *Nuclear perfusion imaging at rest and with stress show a dilated LV with a large inferoposterior wall fixed perfusion abnormality.* Abbreviation: *LV, left ventricle.*

(A)

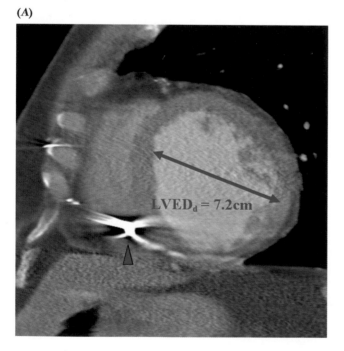

(B)

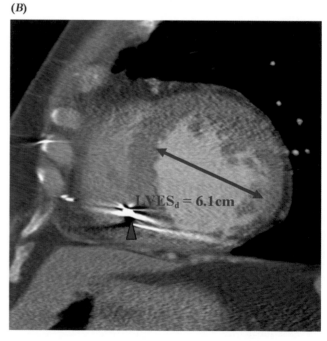

Figure 6.8 *End-diastolic (**A**) and end-systolic (**B**) short-axis frames generated with CT angiography show LV dilatation and systolic dysfunction. Note the tip of the ICD lead (arrowhead) causing metal artifact. The scarred posterior and inferior wall segments are thinned both in diastole and in systole.* Abbreviations: *LV, left ventricle; LVEDd, left ventricular end-diastolic diameter; LVESd, left ventricular end-systolic diameter.*

HYPERTROPHIC CARDIOMYOPATHY

CLINICAL CASE 5

A 58-year-old male smoker presented for evaluation of dyspnea and nonsustained ventricular tachycardia. Physical examination was notable for a systolic ejection murmur at the left sternal border that augmented with standing. Echocardiography showed septal hypertrophy (**Fig. 6.9**).

Multiplanar reformatted CTA images demonstrated marked asymmetric septal hypertrophy as well as systolic anterior motion of the mitral valve (**Fig. 6.10**).

Cardiac catheterization confirmed the diagnosis of hypertrophic obstructive cardiomyopathy with a 30 mmHg gradient along the left ventricular outflow tract (**Fig. 6.11**).

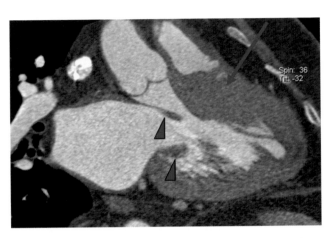

Figure 6.10 *CT angiography data reformatted in the three-chamber plane, demonstrating marked asymmetric hypertrophy of the interventricular septum* (arrow). *Also note thickening of the mitral valve leaflets* (arrowheads).

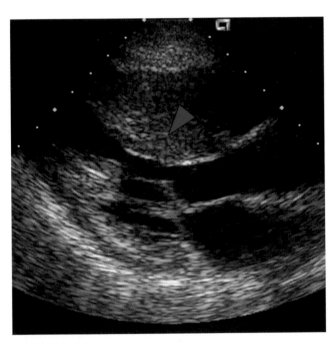

Figure 6.9 *Parasternal long-axis echocardiographic image demonstrates asymmetric septal hypertrophy* (arrowhead).

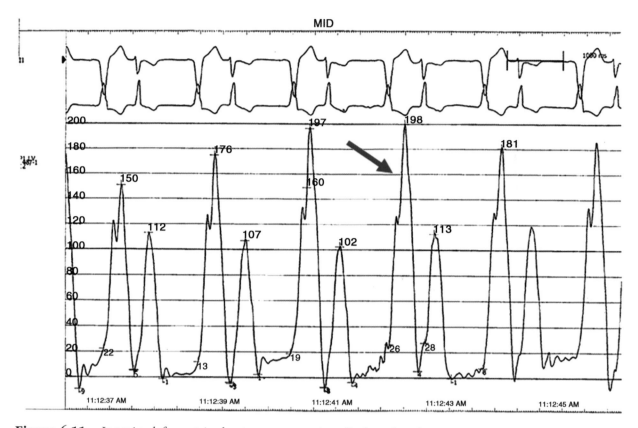

Figure 6.11 *Invasive left ventricular pressure tracing displayed with concurrent electrocardiographic recordings shows the characteristic finding in patients with hypertrophic obstructive cardiomyopathy, namely, postextrasystolic accentuation of the intracavitary gradient* (arrow) *due to reduced volume in the LV cavity.* Abbreviation: *LV, left ventricle.*

DILATED CARDIOMYOPATHY

CLINICAL CASE 6

A 43-year-old female presented to the emergency department with chest pain and shortness of breath. Serial cardiac enzymes and ECGs were negative for acute coronary syndrome. Coronary CTA provided excellent visualization of the coronary tree, which was free of disease (**Fig. 6.12**). However, reformatted multiphase image review identified moderate LV systolic dysfunction, with an LV EF of 35% (**Fig. 6.13**). This was confirmed with invasive angiography and she was initiated on an appropriate medical regimen for dilated cardiomyopathy.

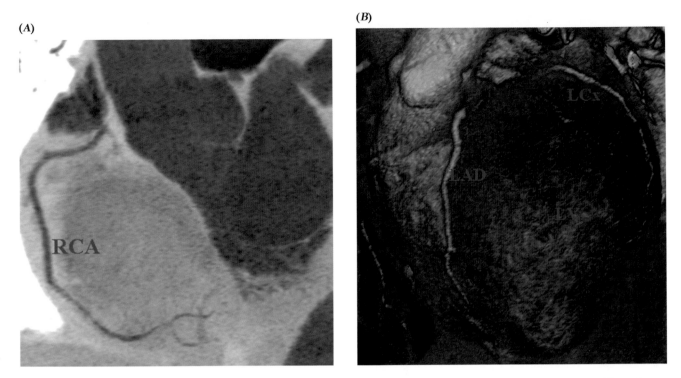

Figure 6.12 *Both right (**A**) and left (**B**) coronary arteries in a patient with chest pain and shortness of breath are free of atherosclerotic disease by CT angiography.* Abbreviations: *RCA, right coronary artery; LCA, left coronary artery; LCx, left circumflex coronary artery; LV, left ventricle.*

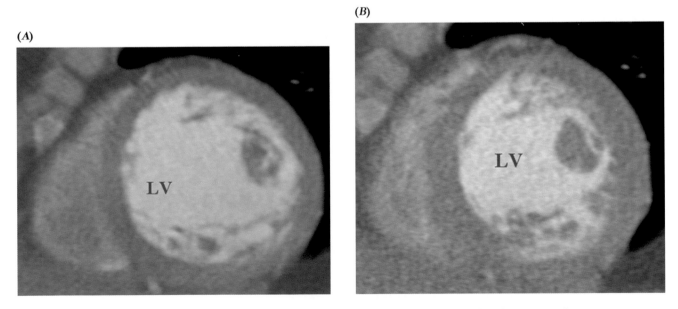

Figure 6.13 *End-diastolic (**A**) and end-systolic (**B**) frames reformatted to the short-axis plane in a patient with shortness of breath, chest pain, and normal coronary arteries by CT angiography demonstrate global left ventricular systolic dysfunction, ejection fraction 35%.*

VENTRICULAR NONCOMPACTION

CLINICAL CASE 7

An 18-year-old male diagnosed with "idiopathic" dilated cardiomyopathy presented for evaluation of chest pain and shortness of breath. CTA showed severe dilatation and severe systolic dysfunction of the LV: LVEDV 380 mL, LVESV 311 mL, and LV EF 18%. The coronary arteries were normal. The morphology of the LV endocardium had poor definition of the endocardial surface and papillary muscles with prominent myocardial trabeculations (**Fig. 6.14**) consistent with the diagnosis of ventricular noncompactation.

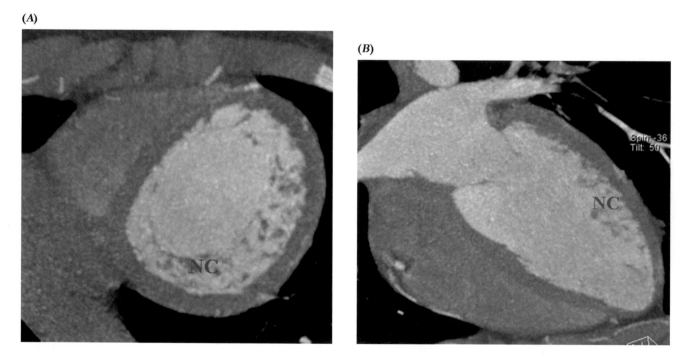

Figure 6.14 *Short-axis (**A**) and horizontal long-axis (**B**) reformatted CT angiography images show an ill-defined noncompacted (NC) LV endocardial surface, consistent with the diagnosis of ventricular noncompaction defined as excessive trabeculations and intertrabecular recesses of the endocardium.*

LV THROMBUS AND PERFUSION DEFECT

CLINICAL CASE 8

A 61-year-old male with remote myocardial infarction accompanied by stroke presented for routine follow-up. He had been taking systemic anticoagulation after his initial event, but had stopped such a few years ago because he was feeling well and disliked the inconveniences associated with taking warfarin. CTA showed a thin, akinetic septum and apex consistent with prior infarct, diffuse atherosclerotic CAD, and moderate segmental contraction abnormality with LV dilatation: LVEDV 245 mL, LVESV 159 mL, and LV EF 35%. Review of reformatted images in short- and long-axis planes revealed thrombus in the left ventricular apex (**Fig. 6.15**) that was also seen with DME-CMR (**Fig. 6.16**).

(A)

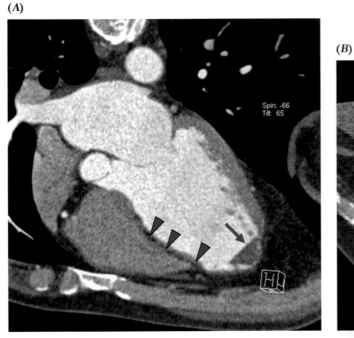

(B)

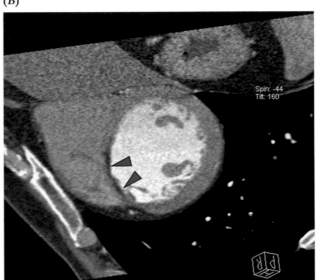

(C)

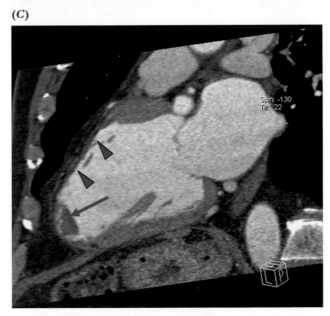

Figure 6.15 *Reformatted CT angiography images in the horizontal long axis (**A**), short axis (**B**), and vertical long axis (**C**) planes show apical thrombus* (arrow) *as well as perfusion abnormality* (arrowheads) *in the thinned anterior wall, septum, and apex.*

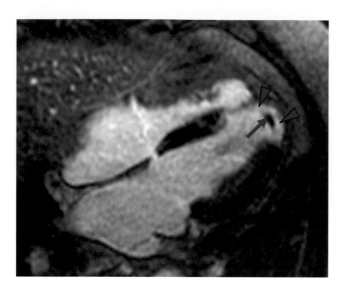

Figure 6.16 *Delayed post–gadolinium imaging optimized for LV scar imaging with cardiac magnetic resonance readily identifies apical thrombus* (arrow) *as a black area adjacent to transmural hyperenhancement or scar* (arrowheads). *Abbreviation: LV, left ventricle.*

VENTRICULAR ASSIST DEVICES

CLINICAL CASE 9

A 40-year-old male with history of transposition of great arteries status post Mustard repair had developed progressive failure of the systemic right ventricle, prompting placement of a ventricular assist device. CTA showed appropriate position of the inflow and outflow cannulae (**Fig. 6.17**).

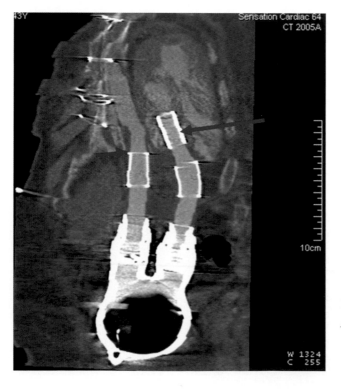

Figure 6.17 *Multiplanar reformatted image showing placement of a ventricular assist device with the inflow cannula drawing blood from the decompressed systemic right ventricle* (arrow) *and the outflow cannula connecting to the aorta* (short arrow).

CLINICAL CASE 10

A 49-year-old male with ischemic cardiomyopathy developed profoundly limiting symptoms due to low cardiac output. He successfully underwent placement of a left ventricular assist device, placement of which was confirmed with CTA (**Fig. 6.18**).

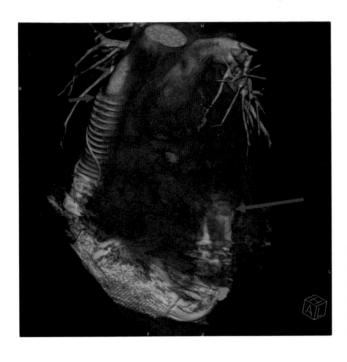

Figure 6.18 *Volume rendering of CT angiography data demonstrates an intact left ventricular assist device, with the inflow cannula emanating from the LV apex* (arrow) *and the outflow cannula connecting to the ascending aorta* (short arrow). Abbreviation: *LV, left ventricle.*

CLINICAL PEARLS

- Dyspnea suspected to be coronary in origin can be assessed with CTA, particularly with limited ability to exercise or contraindication to receiving a vasodilating stress agent.
- CTA provides both coronary and left ventricular assessment in patients with LV dysfunction of unknown etiology, helping to distinguish between ischemic and nonischemic cardiomyopathy.
- Left ventricular volumes, EF, and cavity dimensions can be quantified with CTA, and results are comparable to those obtained with other cardiac imaging modalities.
- Noncompaction of the LV, defined as excessive trabeculations and intertrabecular recesses of the endocardium, and the concomitant ventricular dysfunction are readily demonstrated with CTA.

- CTA identifies myocardial scar or resting ischemia as regions of subendocardial hypoenhancement, providing additional functional information in patients undergoing CT coronary angiography.
- Recognition of LV dysfunction with CTA multiphase imaging may prompt further assessment with CMR. CMR can define the extent of fibrosis and microvascular disease. Myocardial hyperenhancement may represent infarct scar, fibrosis, or infiltrative processes; lack of hyperenhancement indicated viable myocardium and can predict response to medical therapy or revascularization.
- LV thrombus can be identified with CTA, just as with delayed post–gadolinium CMR imaging.

- Limited acoustic windows due to obesity and lung hyperinflation can limit the ability to visualize the heart adequately with echo-cardiography, both of which are less limiting for CTA.
- Multiphase reformatted images in horizontal long-axis planes in patients with hypertrophic cardiomyopathy with CTA allows for recognition of asymmetric septal hypertrophy as well as systolic anterior motion of the anterior mitral valve leaflet.
- Patients with hypertrophic cardiomyopathy have increased incidence of bridging coronary artery segments, which can also be defined using CTA (see Chapter 3).
- Ventricular assist devices may be visualized with excellent detail using CTA, allowing confirmation of placement of the inflow and outflow cannulae. CTA also allows assessment of LV function in patients with implanted pacemakers and ICDs, providing an alternative to CMR.

Chapter 7   The right ventricle

As with imaging of any cardiac chamber, computed tomography imaging of the right ventricle (RV) requires optimal timing of contrast arrival in the RV for good endocardial delineation. Appropriate timing can be gauged by first performing a test bolus with 10 to 20 cc of contrast and determining the time to peak signal intensity within the pulmonary artery. Since contrast fills the RV early with typical venous injection, one might consider increasing the delay to avoid excess residual contrast in the SVC during the helical acquisition. While typical timing for left ventricle (LV) opacification is too late for good right heart visualization, a compromise may be achieved with a delay intermediate between the times to peak signal intensity in the pulmonary artery and in the aorta. Some advocate injecting a mix of contrast and saline simultaneously after the contrast bolus injection (instead of a saline-only flush) to achieve both left and right heart opacification. Regularity of rhythm and selection of the optimal phase for image reconstruction remain important; as with LV systolic function quantification, functional assessment of the right heart requires multiphase reformats covering the cardiac cycle for cine imaging.

Right heart questions often require assessment of the RV outflow tract, pulmonic valve, and the pulmonary arteries as well; this is particularly true in many forms of congenital heart disease with right heart involvement such as tetralogy of Fallot. Arrhythmogenic right ventricular dysplasia/cardiomyopathy can be accurately diagnosed with CT angiography (CTA) using the protocol described above, particularly given the clear distinction of fat from myocardium by Hounsfield unit (HU) interrogation and the ability to recognize regional RV wall motion abnormalities. Modalities such as echocardiography and SPECT imaging have difficulties in volumetric visualization of RV inflow, RV outflow, the pulmonic valve, and pulmonary arteries. For these reasons as well as increasing the use of implantable devices that preclude magnetic resonance imaging, volumetric cardiac CT and the ability to reformat the axial data set in any plane is a tremendous addition to the right heart assessment armamentarium.

NORMAL RV

CLINICAL CASE 1

A 56-year-old female underwent coronary CTA for evaluation of chest pain. Coronary arteries were normal, and multiplanar reformatted images showed normal RV size and systolic function. The RV can be assessed in standard short-axis and long-axis planes, as well as in planes optimized to visualize various segments of the RV myocardium, such as the RV inflow view obtainable from the LV horizontal long-axis plane (**Fig. 7.1**).

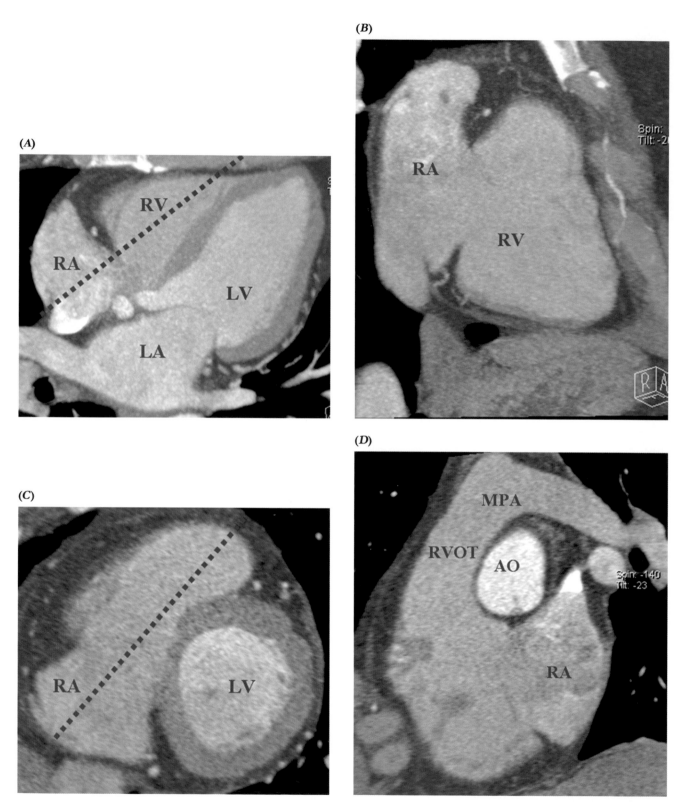

Figure 7.1 *The right ventricle can be visualized in standard planes such as the horizontal long-axis and short-axis planes (**A**, **C**) or in right ventricular inflow (**B**) and outflow (**D**) planes derived as shown with the dotted lines.* Abbreviations: *RA, right atrium; RV, right ventricle; LV, left ventricle; LA, left atrium; RVOT, right ventricular outflow tract; MPA, main pulmonary artery; AO, aorta.*

ABNORMAL RV

CLINICAL CASE 2

A 68-year-old male with repaired tetralogy of Fallot and free pulmonic insufficiency as well as coronary artery disease underwent coronary CTA for assessment of both the coronary arteries and right ventricular size and function quantification.

Coronary CTA showed severely enlarged RV (**Figs. 7.2–7.4**) with moderate global systolic dysfunction: RV ejection fraction (EF) 39%. There was mild global systolic dysfunction of the LV, in the presence of an abnormal septal bounce secondary to right ventricular volume overload.

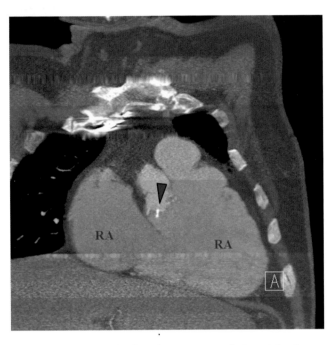

Figure 7.2 *Marked enlargement of the right heart in a patient with repaired tetralogy of Fallot and free pulmonary insufficiency. Also note partial visualization of a calcified ventricular septal defect patch in this plane* (arrowhead). Abbreviations: *RA, right atrium; RV, right ventricle.*

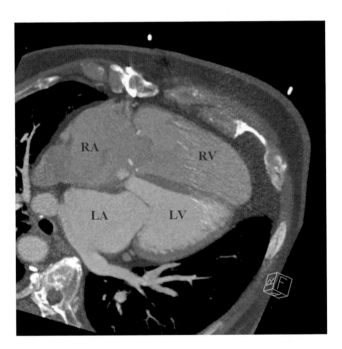

Figure 7.3 *A horizontal long-axis reformatted image in a patient with right heart enlargement due to free pulmonary insufficiency in the setting of repaired tetralogy of Fallot. Abbreviations: RA, right atrium; RV, right ventricle; LA, left atrium; LV, left ventricle.*

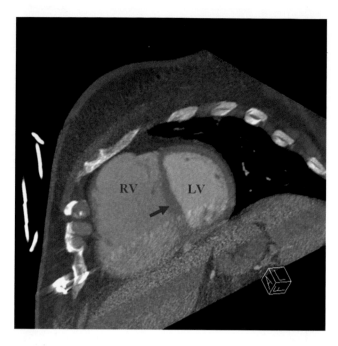

Figure 7.4 *A short-axis view of the dilated RV. Note the flattened septum due to RV volume overload* (arrow). Abbreviation: *RV, right ventricle.*

ARRHYTHMOGENIC RIGHT VENTRICULAR CARDIOMYOPATHY

CLINICAL CASE 3

A 27-year-old female with syncope status post pacemaker placement presented for evaluation of recurrent syncope and ventricular arrhythmias on electrocardiographic monitoring. CTA showed normal coronary arteries; RV morphology was consistent with arrhythmogenic right ventricular cardiomyopathy (ARVC, **Fig. 7.5**).

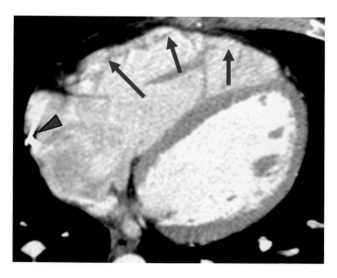

Figure 7.5 *Axial image in a patient with a pacemaker* (arrowhead) *and recurrent syncope in the setting of ventricular arrhythmias demonstrates the scalloped appearance of the RV myocardium* (arrows) *in addition to segmental contraction abnormality of the RV, consistent with the diagnosis of ARVC.* Abbreviation: *RV, right ventricle.*

RIGHT HEART DEVICES

CLINICAL CASE 4

A 58-year-old male with ischemic cardiomyopathy had a right heart pacemaker/defibrillator implanted and underwent coronary CTA.

This showed severe LV systolic dysfunction with marked dyssynchrony of the septum (**Fig. 7.6**). On the basis of these findings, he underwent revision to a biventricular pacing device. Repeat CTA demonstrated that three pacer leads were visualized with CS lead tip visualized at the basal posterolateral wall of the LV (**Figs. 7.7** and **7.8**).

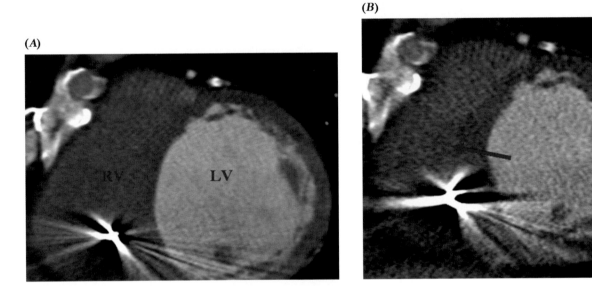

(A)

(B)

Figure 7.6 *CTA-reformatted images in the short-axis plane at end-diastole (**A**) and end-systole (**B**) demonstrate dyssynchronous motion of the interventricular septum relative to the lateral wall during contraction* (arrows indicating septal and lateral wall motion). *Note the artifact due to the RV pacemaker lead.* Abbreviation: *RV, right ventricle.*

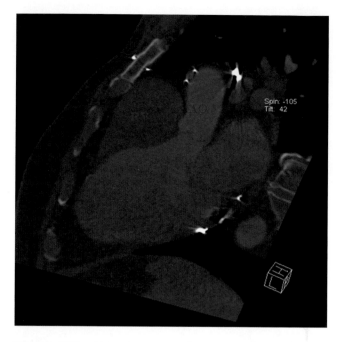

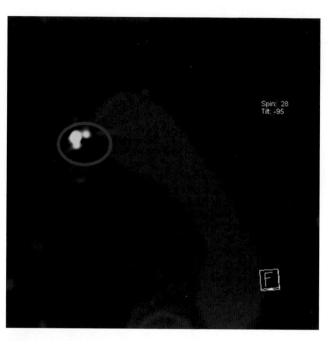

Figure 7.7 *Repeat computed tomography angiography after revision of the implantable device now shows the tip of an LV lead over the basal posterior wall of the LV* (arrow). Abbreviations: *LV, left ventricle; RV, right ventricle; AO, ascending aorta; LA, left atrium.*

Figure 7.8 *Axial computed tomography angiography image after device revision shows three leads in cross-section in the superior vena cava* (encircled).

CLINICAL CASE 5

A 36-year-old female with complex cyanotic heart disease presented for follow-up evaluation with CTA. This showed multiple retained epicardial pacemaker leads (**Fig. 7.9**), normal origin and proximal course of coronary arteries, native pulmonary valve seen below the level of the main pulmonary artery band, dilated LV with mild global systolic dysfunction (EF 45%).

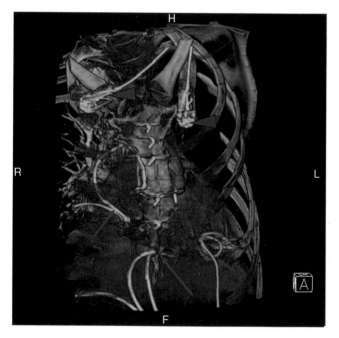

Figure 7.9 *Multiple retained epicardial leads* (arrows) *in a patient with complex congenital heart disease. Note that these are within the chest cavity overlying the heart and are distinct from the surface electrodes* (arrowheads).

CLINICAL CASE 6

A 35-year-old male with connective tissue disease status post prior aortic valve replacement required reoperation for severe aortic stenosis and insufficiency. CTA was performed to define the coronary artery anatomy, which was normal. The presence of a Swan–Ganz (SG) catheter is appreciated (**Fig. 7.10**).

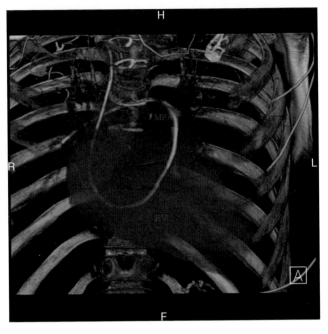

Figure 7.10 *An SG hemodynamic catheter is seen in the superior vena cava traversing the RA, RV, and MPA to reach its destination in the right pulmonary artery.* Abbreviations: *SG, Swan–Ganz; RA, right atrium; RV, right ventricle; MPA, main pulmonary artery.*

CLINICAL PEARLS

- Careful reformatting of volumetric CTA data allows reconstruction of images in optimal planes to allow visualization of right heart chambers.
- RV volumes and EF can be quantified with CTA assuming adequate contrast in the right heart, which may require modification of the contrast delivery protocol.
- CTA allows noninvasive diagnosis of ARVC, a potentially lethal cause of ventricular arrhythmias and syncope. Diagnosis of ARVC may not be feasible with cardiac magnetic resonance (MR) imaging in patients with MR incompatible devices such as defibrillators placed for ventricular tachycardia. In these patients, CTA may demonstrate fibrofatty replacement (low HU), aneurysms, and RV systolic dysfunction (4D-cine CT).
- Right heart devices such as pacemakers, defibrillators, and Swan-Ganz catheters can be visualized with CTA. Despite metal artifact, multidetector CTA can identify the location of such devices, particularly the location of resynchronization leads.
- Dyssynchronous cardiac contraction such as that due to right ventricular pacing can be appreciated with multiphase CTA imaging.

Chapter 8   Valvular heart disease

AORTIC STENOSIS

CLINICAL CASE 1

A 59-year-old male with hyperlipidemia and aortic stenosis that was determined to be mild by invasive catheterization one year ago presented for evaluation of progressive dyspnea. Results of serial echocardiography were incongruous with respect to valvular disease severity and patient symptoms. To define possible etiologies of his dyspnea including more severe aortic stenosis versus atherosclerotic coronary artery disease (CAD), he was referred for CT angiography (CTA).

This showed a calcified, trileaflet aortic valve (**Fig. 8.1**), with direct planimetry resulting in a valve area of 1.2 cm², mild nonobstructive calcified plaque in the left anterior descending coronary artery (LAD) (**Fig. 8.2**), and normal left ventricle (LV) size and systolic function with ejection fraction (EF) 62%. Aortic root dimensions were within normal limits.

(A)

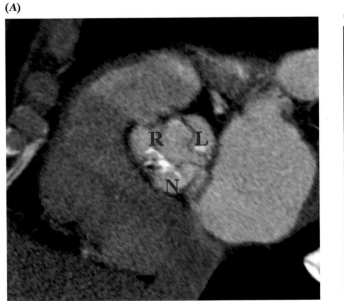

(B)

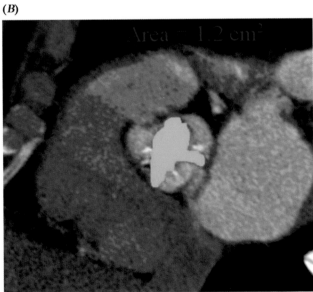

Figure 8.1   (A) En face multiplanar reformatted view of the aortic valve shows focal calcification and a trileaflet structure with mild stenosis by direct planimetry. (B) Coronary cusps are labeled as right (R), left (L), and noncoronary (N).

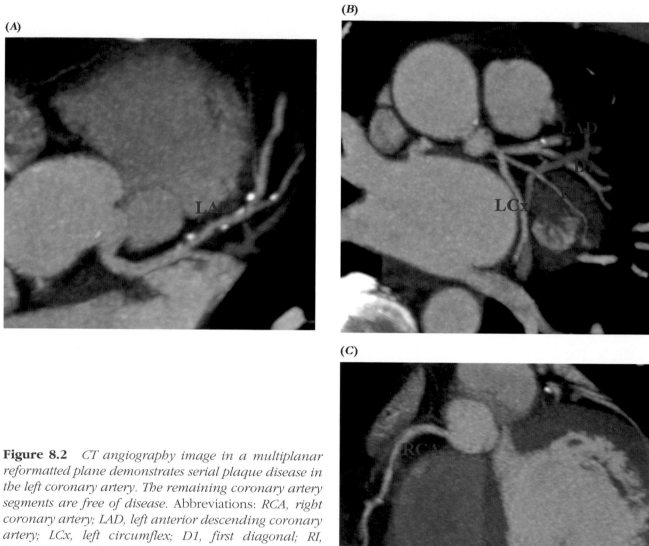

Figure 8.2 *CT angiography image in a multiplanar reformatted plane demonstrates serial plaque disease in the left coronary artery. The remaining coronary artery segments are free of disease.* Abbreviations: *RCA, right coronary artery; LAD, left anterior descending coronary artery; LCx, left circumflex; D1, first diagonal; RI, Ramus Intermedius.*

CLINICAL CASE 2

A 35 year-old female with a history of subaortic membrane presented for follow-up evaluation of the subaortic region, aortic valve, and aorta with CTA. The subaortic membrane was well visualized with both volume rendering and multiplanar reformatted (MPR) image review (**Figs. 8.3** and **8.4**).

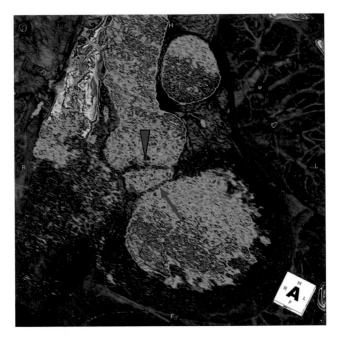

Figure 8.3 *Volume rendering of the left ventricle and the aorta in an oblique coronal plane shows a subaortic membrane* (arrow) *just below the aortic valve* (arrowhead).

(A)   **(B)**

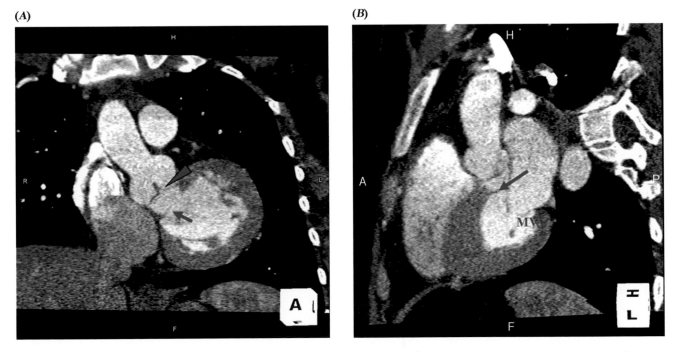

Figure 8.4 *Oblique coronal (**A**) and sagittal (**B**) multiplanar reformatted images demonstrate a subaortic membrane* (arrow). Abbreviation: *MV, mitral valve.*

BICUSPID AORTIC VALVE

CLINICAL CASE 3

A 34-year-old male with aortic coarctation presented for CTA to evaluate the aorta, coronary arteries, and aortic valve. MPR imaging readily demonstrated the aortic valve to be bicuspid (**Fig. 8.5**).

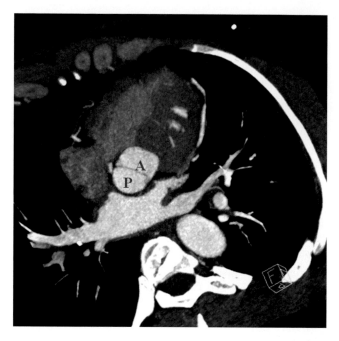

Figure 8.5   *Multiplanar reformatted CT angiography image reformatted in diastole to visualize the closed aortic valve* en face *demonstrates a bicuspid aortic valve.* Abbreviations: *A, anterior leaflet; P, posterior leaflet.*

MITRAL ANNULAR CALCIFICATION

CLINICAL CASE 4

A 48-year-old male with hyperlipidemia, hypertension, family history of premature atherosclerosis, and hepatic cirrhosis with severe functional limitation was seen for pre–liver transplantation evaluation. CTA was performed to assess for CAD. This showed dilated proximal pulmonary vasculature without gross proximal thromboembolic disease, moderate right ventricle enlargement with preserved systolic function, and normal LV size with hyperdynamic systolic function (EF 70%). There was mild mitral annular calcification and angiographically normal coronary arteries (**Fig. 8.6**).

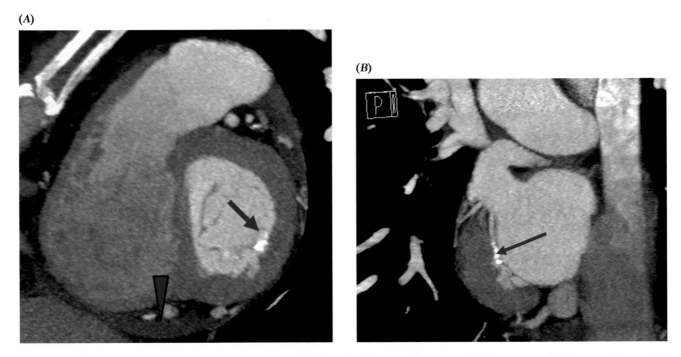

(A)

(B)

Figure 8.6 *Short axis (**A**) and posterior coronal (**B**) multiplanar reformatted CT angiography images show mild focal mitral annular calcification* (arrow) *as well as a small amount of pericardial fluid* (arrowheads). *Note that in the coronal plane, the linear appearance of the mitral annular calcification should not be confused with coronary calcification.*

MITRAL VALVE PROLAPSE

CLINICAL CASE 5

A 52-year-old male with a family history of premature CAD presented for evaluation of substernal chest pain and was referred for coronary CTA. This demonstrated separate ostia of the left circumflex and LAD directly from the left aortic sinus of Valsalva along with aneurysm of the aorta (aortic sinuses measured 49 mm), isolated plaque disease of the coronary arteries (proximal/mid-LAD), prolapse of the anterior mitral valve leaflet (**Fig. 8.7**), and normal left ventricular systolic function. Echocardiography confirmed the diagnosis of mitral valve prolapse (**Fig. 8.8**) in this patient with connective tissue disease.

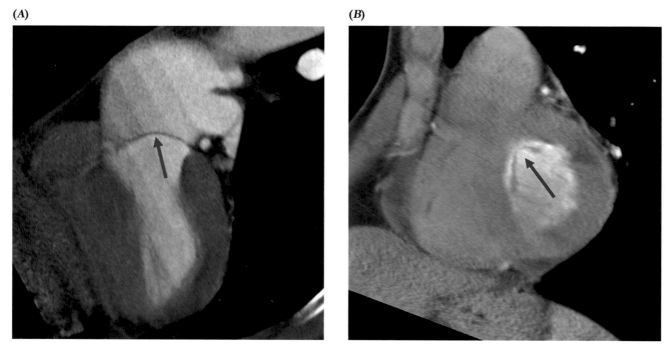

(A)   (B)

Figure 8.7   *CT angiography images reformatted in the vertical long axis (**A**) and basal short axis (**B**) planes demonstrate prolapse of the anterior leaflet of the mitral valve* (arrow).

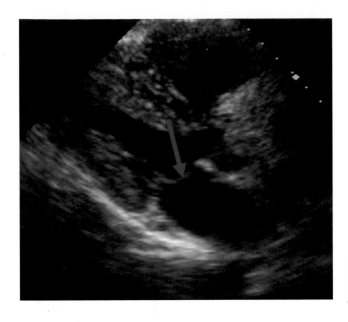

Figure 8.8 *Parasternal long axis view obtained with echocardiography confirms anterior mitral valve leaflet prolapse* (arrow).

SYSTOLIC ANTERIOR MOTION OF THE MITRAL VALVE

CLINICAL CASE 6

A 58-year-old male smoker with hypertrophic cardiomyopathy underwent multiphase cardiac CTA (see also Chapter 3). MPR CTA images demonstrated marked asymmetric septal hypertrophy as well as systolic anterior motion of the mitral valve (**Fig. 8.9**).

(A)

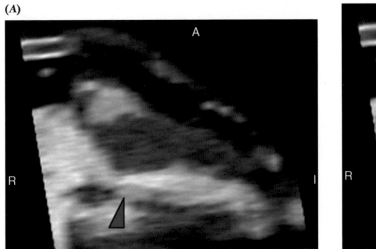

(B)

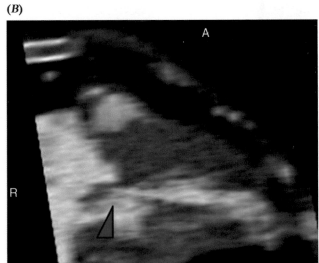

Figure 8.9 *Serial systolic frames (**A** and **B**) demonstrate systolic anterior motion of the mitral valve* (arrowheads).

MITRAL STENOSIS

CLINICAL CASE 7

A 40-year-old woman sought medical attention for nine months of progressive exertional dyspnea. Cardiac auscultation demonstrated a low-pitched diastolic rumble and mitral opening snap. Echocardiography confirmed moderate mitral valve stenosis. She subsequently underwent cardiac CTA, which showed coronary arteries free of disease. CTA also demonstrated marked thickening of the mitral valve leaflets and subvalvular structures without calcification (**Fig. 8.10**). While not the primary indication for CTA in this case, review of MPR images as well as multiphase data allowed calculation of a mitral valvuloplasty score (American and Canadian Societies of Echocardiography). This score rates leaflet mobility, valve thickening, calcification, and subvalvular thickening, each on a 0-to-4 scale. A score greater than 8 portends poor results with valvuloplasty; this patient's score by echocardiography as well as CTA was 8, and she was referred for valve replacement surgery.

(A)

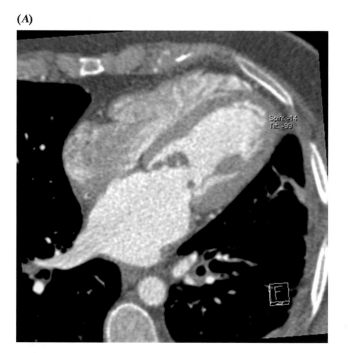

(B)

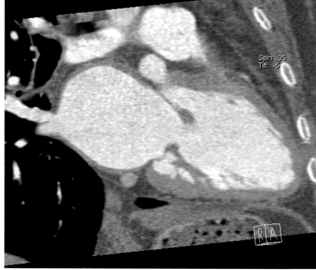

Figure 8.10   (Continued)

(C)

(D)

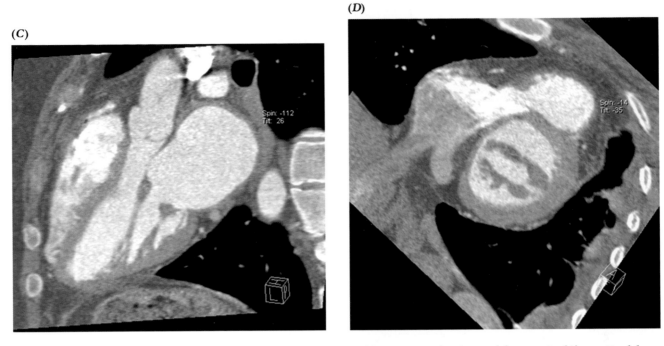

Figure 8.10 (Continued) *Maximum intensity projection CT images in horizontal long-axis (**A**), vertical long axis (**B**), three-chamber (**C**), and basal short axis (**D**) planes demonstrate marked thickening of the mitral valve apparatus in a patient with rheumatic mitral stenosis. Notable is the lack of calcification of the bulky leaflet deposits, which is in contrast to advanced calcific mitral stenosis. The degree of leaflet mobility can be assessed by reviewing the dynamic multiphase CT images.*

PROSTHETIC HEART VALVES

CLINICAL CASE 8

A 53-year-old male with a history of mechanical mitral valve replacement, hypertension, hyperlipidemia, and family history of CAD presented for evaluation of intermittent sharp, left-sided chest pain. CTA showed no CAD and intact bileaflet tilting disk mitral valve prosthesis (**Fig. 8.11**).

(A)

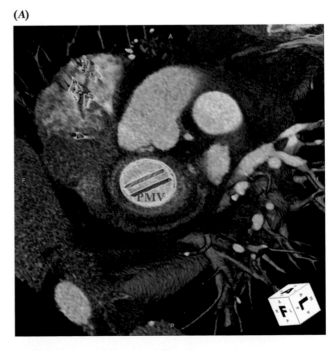

Figure 8.11 (Continued)

(B)

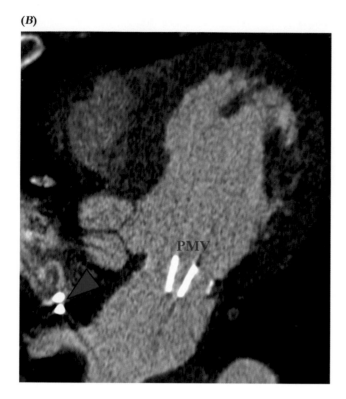

Figure 8.11 (Continued) *Volume-rendered short axis (**A**) and multiplanar reformatted long axis (**B**) views of a bileaflet tilting disk mitral valve prosthesis. Also note in (**B**) two pacing leads seen in cross-section in the right atrium* (arrowhead). Abbreviation: *PMV, prosthetic mitral valve.*

CLINICAL CASE 9

A 68-year-old female smoker with prior aortic valve replacement presented for follow-up evaluation. CTA demonstrated an intact pericardial tissue aortic bioprosthesis (**Fig. 8.12**).

(A)

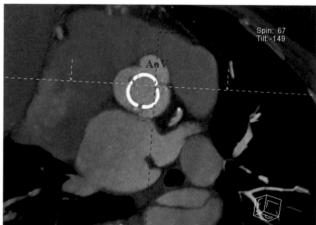

Figure 8.12 (Continued)

(B)

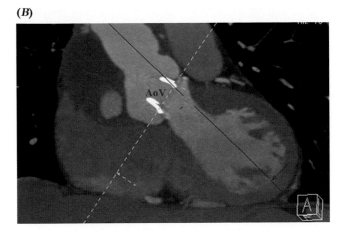

Figure 8.12 (Continued) *Multiplanar reformatted images demonstrate various views of a pericardial tissue bioprosthetic AoV.* Abbreviation: *AoV, aortic valve.*

CLINICAL CASE 10

A 30-year-old male with a history of prosthetic replacement of a stenotic bicuspid aortic valve presented for routine follow-up evaluation. Due to third degree atrioventricular block after valve replacement, he required dual chamber pacemaker placement.

Cardiac CTA showed an intact bileaflet tilting disk in the aortic position (**Fig. 8.13**), normal dimensions of the arch and descending thoracic aorta, normal systolic function of the LV, the dual chamber pacemaker, and multiple retained epicardial pacemaker leads.

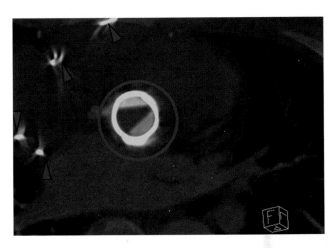

Figure 8.13 *Bileaflet tilting disk aortic valve prosthesis* (circle) *by CT angiography multiplanar reformatting. Also note multiple pacemaker lead artifacts* (arrowheads).

CLINICAL CASE 11

A 68-year-old male who had undergone prior mitral valve annuloplasty and three vessel coronary artery bypass grafting presented for follow-up assessment of grafts with CTA. This demonstrated two of three patent grafts, normal LV size and systolic function, and an intact mitral valve annuloplasty ring (**Fig. 8.14**).

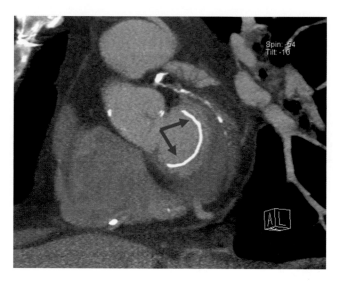

Figure 8.14   *Multiplanar reformatted image in a left anterior oblique plane demonstrates the mitral annuloplasty ring* (arrows).

CLINICAL CASE 12

A 78-year-old patient with history of sick sinus syndrome requiring pacemaker implantation had undergone porcine mitral valve stent replacement and concomitant coronary artery bypass surgery five years prior to current presentation for surgical management of severe calcific aortic valve stenosis. Preoperatively, she was referred for CTA that showed all four bypass grafts to be patent, and left ventricular systolic function to be stable compared to prior assessments (LV EF 41%). The stent valve in the mitral position is shown in **Fig. 8.15**.

(A)

(B)

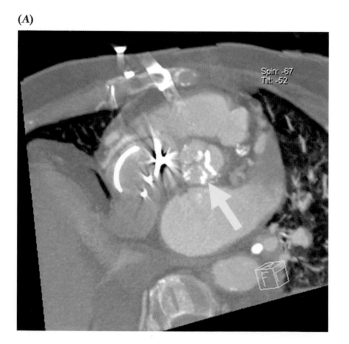
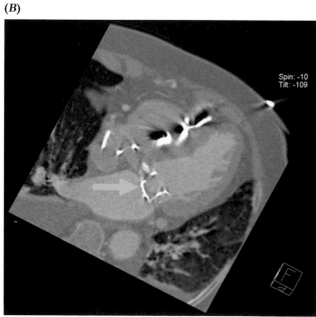

Figure 8.15   (Continued)

(C)

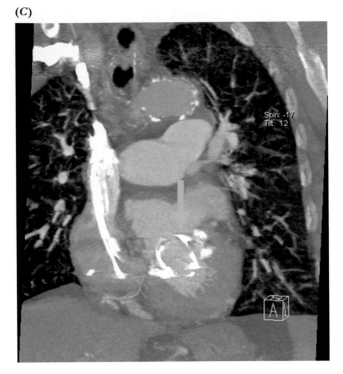

(D)

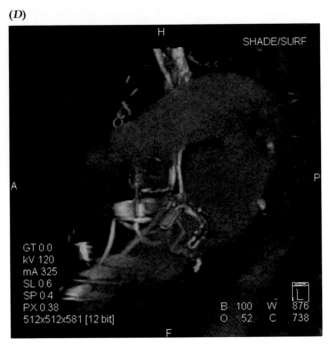

Figure 8.15 (Continued) *(A)* En face *view of the calcified aortic valve leaflets (yellow* arrow*). blue arrows in (B) and (C) indicate the MV prosthesis. (B) shows the MV in a horizontal long axis view and (C) shows the MV prosthesis en face. In (B), the metal loop portion of the stent valve is discernible on the ventricular side of the valve. (D) shows a volume-rendered image of the valve seated within the shadow of the heart; in this format, the three-dimensional structure of the prosthetic valve can be visualized in its entirety. Also note extensive aortic atherosclerosis and considerable artifact from the pacemaker leads (status post multiple revisions).* Abbreviation: *MV, mitral valve.*

CLINICAL CASE 13

A 30-year-old female with a history of congenital atrial septal defect, ventricular septal defect and pulmonary stenosis s/p remote repairs presented with chest pain. Six years prior to current presentation, she had developed severe tricuspid regurgitation and had undergone replacement of the tricuspid valve with a 35mm Hancock porcine valve. Subsequent high-grade conduction system disease prompted pacemaker placement.

Because of chest pain, she was referred for CTA that showed normal coronary arteries. **Fig. 8.16** depicts the tricuspid valve prosthesis by CTA.

A patient with history of St. Jude aortic valve replacement presented with fever and *Staphylococcus aureus* bacteremia. Echocardiography showed severe paravalvular regurgitation. CTA demonstrated a large abscess cavity (**Fig. 8.17**). This finding was confirmed by re-examination via transesophageal echo.

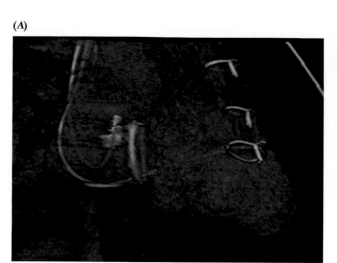

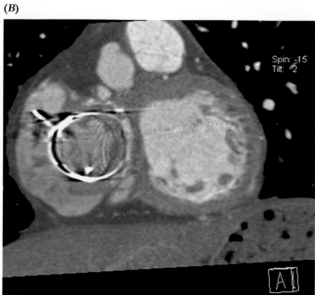

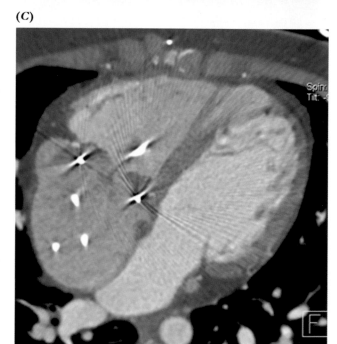

Figure 8.16 (*A*) *Volume rendering of the whole heart and the seat of the tricuspid valve between the right atrium and the right ventricle. Note the two pacemaker leads in the respective right heart chambers. (**B**) En face maximum intensity projection image of the tricuspid valve. (**C**) Horizontal long-axis view of the heart demonstrates the struts of the tricuspid valve prosthesis in a lateral view of the valve.*

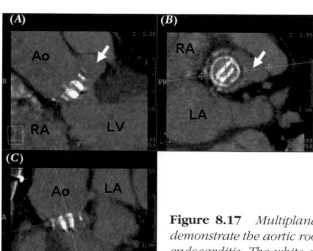

Figure 8.17 *Multiplanar reconstruction planes of the aortic root. Frames (**A–C**) demonstrate the aortic root and sinuses of Valsalva in this patient with prosthetic valve endocarditis. The white arrows in frames (**A**) and (**B**) point to the abscess of the left sinus; this sinus is not visible in the projection shown in frame (**C**). Abbreviations: Ao, aorta; RA, right atrium; LV, left ventricle; LA, left atrium.*

CLINICAL PEARLS

- CTA allows visualization of supravalvular, valvular, and subvalvular pathologies.
- With appropriately selected phase of the cardiac cycle and plane of reformatting, CTA allows for direct valve planimetry in patients with valvular stenosis.
- CTA provides simultaneous coronary artery and cardiac valve assessment, which may be helpful in patients with aortic stenosis being evaluated for valve replacement.
- With imaging of both the aorta and the aortic valve, CTA facilitates selection of surgical technique, e.g., valve replacement alone versus valve and root replacement. Recognition of severe annular calcification, for example, might motivate valve replacement instead of valve repair.
- CTA allows visualization of aortic valve morphology, such as bicuspid versus trileaflet aortic valve. Recognition of a bicuspid aortic valve should prompt evaluation of possible coronary artery anomalies as well as aortic coarctation.
- Simultaneous coronary and valvular assessment is feasible with CTA and may be useful in preoperative assessment of patients, particularly those with stenotic valvular lesions, who may be unable to undergo stress testing.
- In patients being evaluated for CAD with CTA, mitral annular calcification should not be confused with coronary atherosclerosis. Review of the calcified segment in multiple views helps localize the pathology to the annulus.
- In patients with prosthetic heart valves, CTA can identify the type and location of such valves. Multiphase rendering in the appropriate planes can demonstrate valvular motion, although with limited temporal resolution.
- In patients with connective tissue disease, CTA can help identify both valvular heart disease and aortopathy.
- Devices used for valvular repair, such as annuloplasty rings can be evaluated with CTA.

Chapter 9   **Pericardium**

PERICARDIAL EFFUSION

CLINICAL CASE 1

A 44-year-old male with chronic liver disease underwent cardiac computed tomography (CT) imaging for chest pain evaluation. This demonstrated normal coronary arteries as well as a small pericardial effusion (**Fig. 9.1**). Pericardial fluid can be easily differentiated from fat since fat has negative Hounsfield unit (HU) values and tissues and fluid have HU values greater than 0.

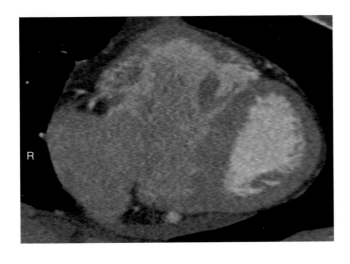

Figure 9.1 *Multiplanar reformatted CT angiography image shows a small pericardial effusion along the inferior wall* (arrow).

PERICARDIAL CALCIFICATION

CLINICAL CASE 2

A 66-year-old male with prior myocardial infarction presented for cardiac magnetic resonance (CMR) examination to define the extent of scar and ischemia.

CMR showed a large mass (**Fig. 9.2**) that appeared to be in the pericardial space impinging upon the inferoposterior wall of the left ventricle (LV) with signal characteristics suggestive of circumferential calcification. There was also focal infero-apical myocardial infarct scar, and overall preserved LV systolic function with ejection fraction (EF) 56%. Because of the superior ability of CT to demonstrate calcification, he was referred for CT angiography (CTA). This showed a 6.4 × 7.2 cm calcified pericardial mass along the inferior/posterior LV and appeared to extend superiorly, invaginating the inferoposterior walls without mitral valve involvement (**Figs. 9.3** and **9.4**). Further patient history revealed remote tuberculosis, confirming the diagnosis of tuberculous pericarditis with subsequent calcification.

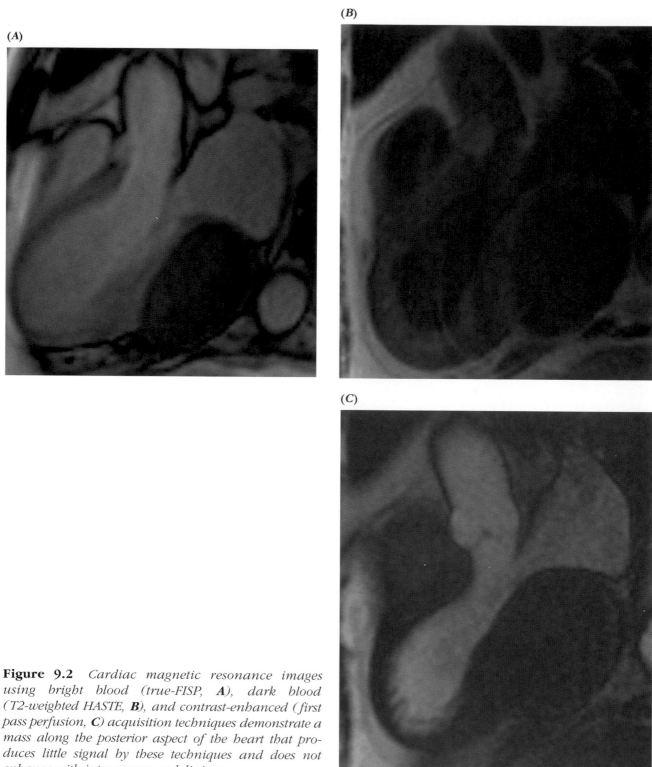

Figure 9.2 *Cardiac magnetic resonance images using bright blood (true-FISP, **A**), dark blood (T2-weighted HASTE, **B**), and contrast-enhanced (first pass perfusion, **C**) acquisition techniques demonstrate a mass along the posterior aspect of the heart that produces little signal by these techniques and does not enhance with intravenous gadolinium.*

(A)

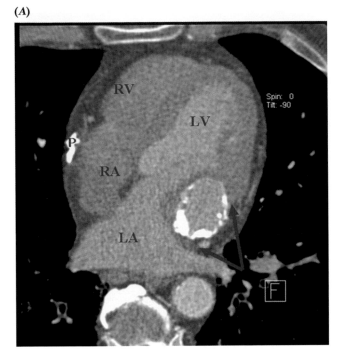

(B)

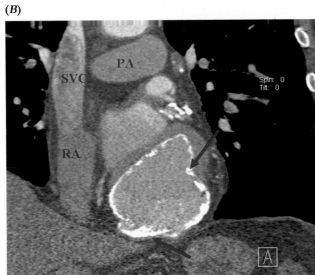

(C)

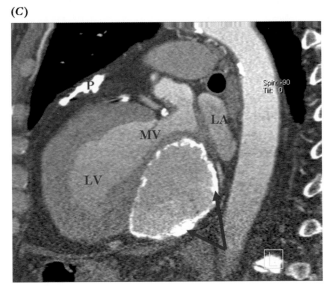

Figure 9.3 *Multiplanar reformatted images show a calcified mass in the pericardial space* (arrows). *Also note other areas of pericardial calcification (P).* Abbreviations: *LA, left atrium; LV, left ventricle; MV, mitral valve; SVC, superior vena cava; RA, right atrium; RV, right ventricle; PA, pulmonary artery.*

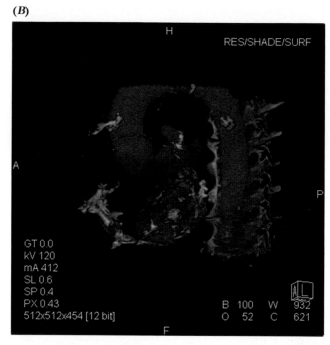

Figure 9.4 *Frame (A) shows the three-dimensional CT angiography data such that calcium is rendered in white. Note the extensive calcified mass overlying and invaginating the left atrium. Frame (B) is a similar volume rendering but with a higher window width (932 vs. 539) and center (621 vs. 254) to emphasize the extent of cardiac calcification.*

CLINICAL CASE 3

A patient with coronary artery disease presented with dyspnea several days after coronary artery bypass surgery. CTA demonstrated a large pericardial effusion (HU = 6.1) as well as air in the pericardial space, i.e., pneumopericardium (**Fig. 9.5**).

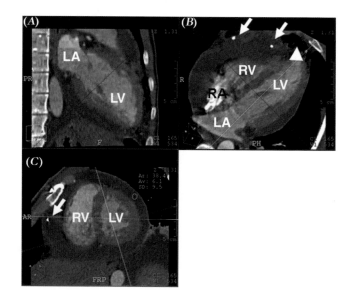

Figure 9.5 *Multiplanar reformatted images in the vertical long axis (A), horizontal long axis (B), and short axis (C) planes show air in the pericardial space (arrowhead) or pneumopericardium. Also note epicardial pacing wires in cross-section (arrows).*

CLINICAL CASE 4

A patient who had undergone recent aortic valve replacement with a bioprosthetic valve presented with pleuritic chest pain. CTA (**Fig. 9.6**) demonstrated thickened parietal and visceral layers of the pericardium and a small pericardial effusion, supporting the diagnosis of pericarditis.

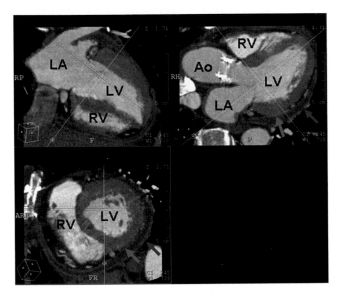

Figure 9.6 *Multiplanar reformatted images of the heart in orthogonal views. All three frames demonstrate the thickening of the visceral and parietal layers of the pericardium* (green arrows indicate visceral pericardium; red arrows indicate parietal pericardium).

CLINICAL CASE 5

A 67-year-old female with recent placement of a biventricular pacemaker presented to the emergency department with sudden onset of neck pain associated with diaphoresis, nausea, and emesis. Because of concern regarding lead-induced myocardial rupture, a chest CT was obtained in the emergency room. This showed a small area of consolidation in the right lung adjacent to the right heart and a questionable pericardial effusion. Coronary CTA performed to evaluate both the coronary arteries and the pericardium revealed a mostly posteriorly located pericardial effusion (**Fig. 9.7**). Perusal of the three-dimensional CTA data set allows assessment of the heart from many perspectives to confirm that there had been no myocardial rupture.

(A)

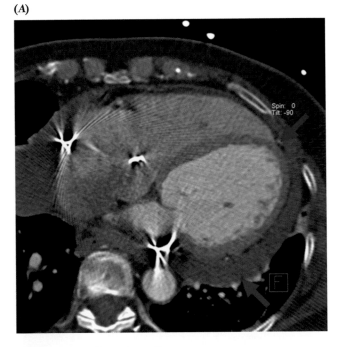

Figure 9.7 (Continued)

(B)

(C)

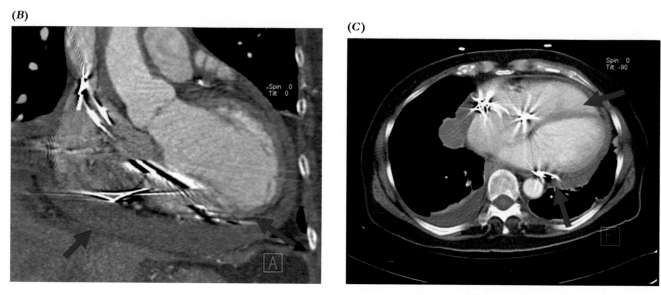

Figure 9.7 (Continued) *Frames (**A**) and (**B**) are multiplanar reconstructed data sets from the same scan done initially at presentation. They reveal a fairly large pericardial effusion with pericardial thickening. Frame (**C**) reveals the same approximate plane as frame about three weeks later. Note the interval improvement of the pericardial thickening and effusion.*

CLINICAL CASE 6

A 31-year-old patient 14 months s/p heart transplant presented with atypical chest pain. CTA showed that the coronary arteries were without disease, but there was a focal area of pericardial thickening and calcification that appeared adherent to the chest wall via extension of the thickened tissue (**Fig. 9.8**).

(A)

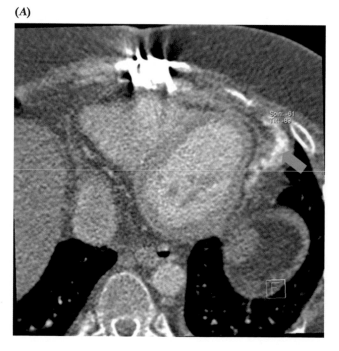

(B)

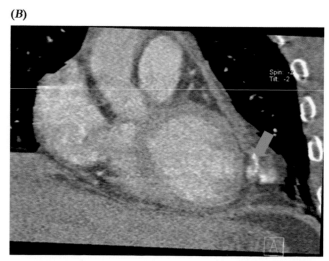

Figure 9.8 (Continued)

(C)

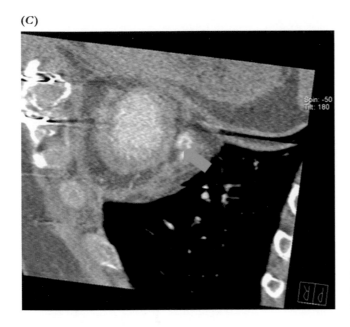

Figure 9.8 (Continued) *Multiplanar reformatted CT angiography images show focal thickening and calcification* (arrows) *of the pericardium that appeared adherent to the chest wall.*

CLINICAL CASE 7

A 42-year-old male presented with symptoms of dyspnea and fatigue, prompting coronary CTA. This revealed focal regions of pericardial calcification (**Fig. 9.9**). There was no significant obstructive coronary disease. Subsequent CMR demonstrated a restrictive filling pattern with a left ventricular EF of 50%.

(A)

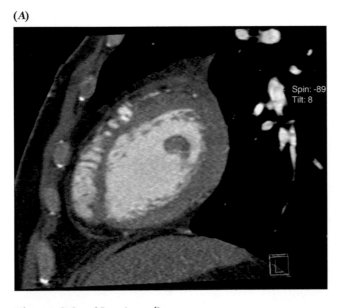

(B)

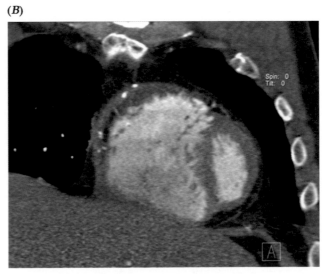

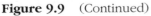

Figure 9.9 (Continued)

(C) *(D)*

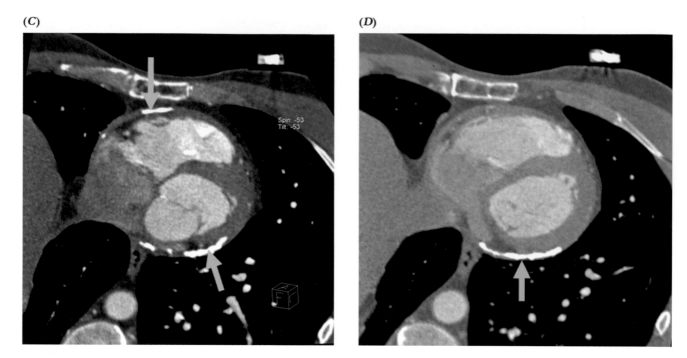

Figure 9.9 (Continued) *Multiplanar reformatted CT angiography images illustrate thickening of the parietal pericardium. Note the focal calcification of the pericardium* (arrows).

CLINICAL PEARLS

- CTA can recognize pericardial thickening and effusions, particularly when the slice thickness is minimized to avoid false-positive assignment of pericardial disease on the basis of partial volume effect.
- CMR is superior to CTA in distinguishing pericardial thickening from effusion.
- CTA is useful in defining calcific pericardial disease, which may be difficult to appreciate with magnetic resonance imaging.
- Patients with connective tissue diseases, infections, or inflammatory conditions presenting with chest pain may have pericardial disease. When concomitant clinical suspicion for coronary artery disease exists, CTA may be a useful modality to address both pericardial and coronary artery questions.
- In patients with calcified or thickened pericardium, cine CT may confirm the presence or absence of a diastolic septal bounce, characteristic of constrictive physiology.

Chapter 10 Aorta

A variety of clinical scenarios, both acute and chronic, may prompt assessment for aortic disease including aneurysm, dissection, atherosclerotic disease and sequelae such as obstructive atheroma and ulceration, grafts, coarctation, aortic stents, and aortic bypass conduits. Multidetector CT angiography (CTA) has revolutionized the diagnosis and management of aortic disease. Decreased scan time, greater spatial resolution, and large anatomic coverage have afforded accurate volumetric assessment of the aorta. A typical aortic CTA protocol involves injection of 100 to 120 mL of iodinated contrast (depending on patient size) at a rate of 3 to 3.5 cc/sec to obtain a scan of the entire aorta, starting from above the arch superiorly to the bifurcation inferiorly. The pitch (table speed for a given gantry rotation time) should be adjusted on the basis of the volume of coverage and the parameters available on the specific system being used. While performing the scan, one must take care not to "outrun" the contrast with the table speed such that image acquisition at a given location coincides with the appearance of contrast at that location. Scan timing for aortic CTA is usually determined using bolus tracking (as opposed to the test bolus delay estimation technique more commonly used in coronary artery CTA). The segment of the aorta for optimal contrast opacification should be identified as the "region of interest" and the bolus tracking should be tailored to the threshold intensity at that region of interest. If the entire aorta is to be imaged, a point at or just below the diaphragm often gives the best average lumen opacification. With bolus tracking, the volume acquisition is triggered to begin once signal intensity in the selected portion of the aorta has reached a certain threshold, such as 100 to 120 Hounsfield units.

Delayed imaging after initial CTA without additional contrast can be immensely helpful in assessing aortic pathology; limiting the coverage to the region of suspected pathology identified from the CTA minimizes additional radiation exposure.

Delayed imaging (or, alternatively, magnetic resonance imaging) can distinguish between slow leak into false lumen and endovascular leak from thrombosed false lumen. The timing of the delayed scan should be within 2 to 5 minutes of the initial first-pass bolus. Localization, classification, and dynamic assessment, when indicated, form the cornerstones of complete aortic assessment, and CTA provides such comprehensive information for serial assessment, intervention planning, and postintervention follow-up.

Careful attention must be paid to the pathology one wishes to identify. For instance, aortic coarctation may involve aortic root dilatation and anomalous coronary arteries. Therefore, one should tailor contrast bolus delivery to opacify the aortic root, coronary arteries, and distal descending thoracic aorta. This may involve moving the region of interest to trigger scanning to a point midway between these areas, or it may entail a slower injection rate than would otherwise be used for imaging any area alone. Breath-hold and electrocardiographic (ECG) gating are essential for CTA of the aortic root. Gated acquisition increases radiation dose but allows multiphase cine reconstructions that can be used to visualize dynamic components of the aortic structure, such as a moving dissection flap.

All modern CT image review workstations allow the simultaneous visualization of a particular segment of the aorta in three orthogonal planes (three-dimensional reformatting of the thin-slice axial data set). Volume rendering techniques are very helpful in providing an overview of the structure of the aorta and associated large branches. However, it is crucial to also carefully inspect the thin-section axial data, making use of multiplanar reformatted images at sites of possible pathology for thorough assessment. Maximum intensity projection (MIP) images may "miss" the false lumen, pseudoaneurysm, thrombus, or ulcerated segments of the vessel wall. Measurements of vessel dimensions should be made in a plane perpendicular to the vessel's lengthwise course, which is infrequently the straight axial plane in patients with significant aortic tortuosity.

CTA allows exquisite assessment of the aorta after surgical or percutaneous intervention, as will be demonstrated in this chapter. One can carefully assess arterial conduits in volume-rendered and MIP formats to demonstrate the relationship between repair materials and native adjacent structures. Erosion, impingement, disassociation, and correct seating of grafts, conduits, and other implanted devices can be assessed quickly and in multiple views from high-resolution data obtained in an 8- to 12-second breath-hold scan. CTA is also particularly useful in assessing reimplanted coronary arteries, often done as part of aortic root and valve surgeries, both from the exterior perspective of the aorta and the coronary arteries as well as from within the contrast-filled coronary lumen.

DISSECTION

CLINICAL CASE 1

A 60-year-old male with hypertension and prior type A aortic dissection treated with tube graft replacement of ascending aorta and resuspension of the aortic valve presented for follow-up evaluation in the setting of chest pain.

Magnetic resonance imaging showed complex residual dissection involving the aortic sinuses below the graft and extending beyond the distal graft anastomosis through the transverse and descending aorta (**Fig. 10.1**).

Because of the concern of residual dissection at the level of the sinuses, the patient underwent CTA (**Fig. 10.2**), which showed complex residual aortic dissection at the level of the sinuses involving the left mainstem coronary artery, an intact short segment of graft in the aortic root, and continuation of the dissection throughout the descending aorta involving the great vessel ostia. The proximal left anterior descending coronary artery had nonobstructive calcific plaque, while the left circumflex and right coronary artery were free of disease; left ventricle (LV) size and systolic function [ejection fraction (EF) 55%] were normal.

Cardiac catheterization verified these findings, and the patient subsequently underwent reoperation including reimplantation of the coronary arteries and great vessels.

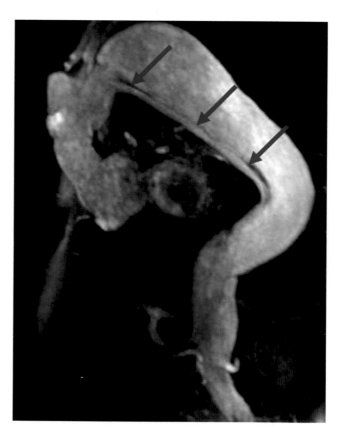

Figure 10.1 *Magnetic resonance angiogram demonstrating a dissection flap in the aorta* (arrows).

(A)

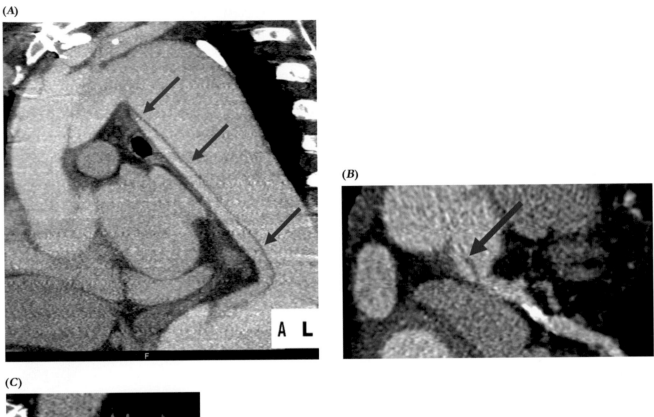

(B)

(C)

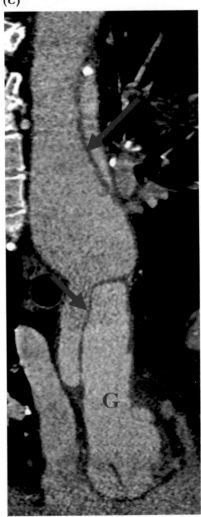

Figure 10.2 *Multiplanar reformatted CT angiography images demonstrate extensive aortic dissection involving the transverse and descending aorta (**A**, arrows) as well as the ostium of the left main coronary artery (**B**, arrow). Rendering of the ascending aorta lengthwise (**C**) shows the relationship of the dissection (arrow) relative to the AAo graft (G). Abbreviation: AAo, ascending aorta.*

CLINICAL CASE 2

A 70-year-old female smoker with long-standing hypertension presented for evaluation of chest pain and dyspnea. CTA showed isolated plaque in the coronary arteries. The thoracic aorta was tortuous with maximum dimension of 4.7 cm and probable leak in the lower descending thoracic aorta, surrounded by fluid collection, which most likely represented blood (**Fig. 10.3**). Surgical consultation was obtained with request for confirmation by invasive aortography. During preparation for the procedure, she experienced sudden severe back pain with hypotension. She was taken emergently to the operating room where she was found to have a ruptured thoracoabdominal aneurysm at the suspected leak site, which was successfully repaired.

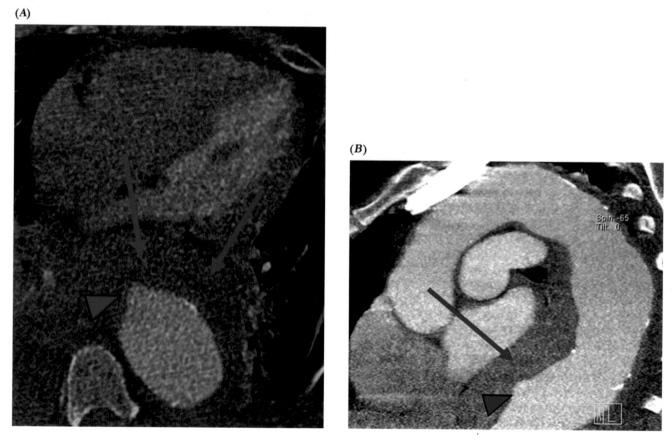

(A)

(B)

Figure 10.3 *Reformatted CT angiography images demonstrate a focal outpouching in a tortuous thoraco-abdominal aorta* (arrowhead) *with extensive collection of periaortic fluid* (arrows), *consistent with leak, which could be further confirmed with five-minute delayed imaging.*

CLINICAL CASE 3

A 68-year-old female smoker with prior type A dissection repair with root replacement and subsequent aortic valve replacement presented one month after her second surgery with a transient episode of chest pain. Echocardiography showed an intact bioprosthetic aortic valve but poor visualization of the recent postoperative root region (**Fig. 10.4**).

CTA showed type A dissection s/p repair and aortic valve replacement. Additionally, there was demonstration of a collection of contrast communicating with the ascending aorta just above noncoronary and just below proximal anastomosis of Hemashield graft, suggestive of leak (**Fig. 10.5**). The patient was referred for transcatheter repair, which was performed successfully. Post-repair CTA demonstrated an intact repair site (**Fig. 10.6**).

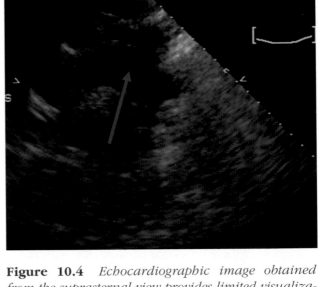

Figure 10.4 *Echocardiographic image obtained from the suprasternal view provides limited visualization of the aortic and graft anatomy* (arrow).

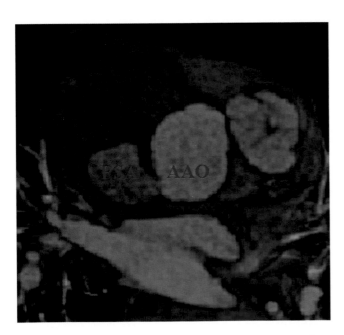

Figure 10.5 *CT angiography demonstrates a collection of contrast outside of but communicating with the AAo, consistent with a PSA.* Abbreviations: *AAo, ascending aorta; PSA, pseudoaneurysm.*

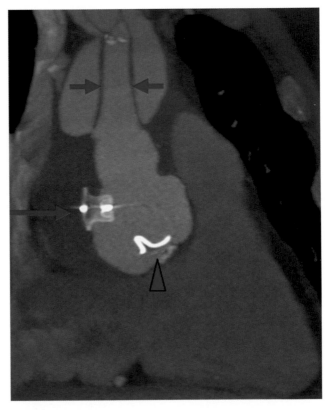

Figure 10.6 *Post-transcatheter repair CT angiography demonstrating an intact occluder device* (arrow). *Note also the struts of the bioprosthetic aortic valve* (arrowhead) *and the dissection* (short arrows) *continuing beyond the aortic root replacement.*

COARCTATION

CLINICAL CASE 4

A 27-year-old white male with aortic coarctation and prior surgical repair presented for evaluation of coronary artery and aortic anatomy, particularly important since prior operative records were unavailable. CTA demonstrated coarctation of the aorta with an intact jump graft from ascending to descending aorta, bicuspid aortic valve, and normal coronary arteries (**Fig. 10.7**).

(A)

(B)

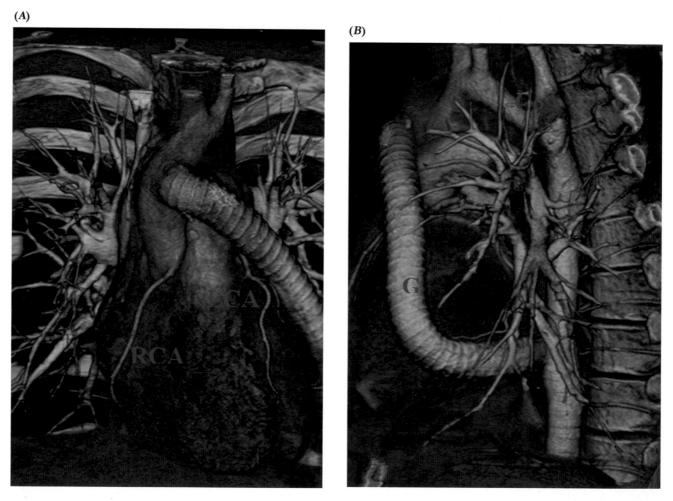

Figure 10.7 *Volume-rendered CT angiography images demonstrate an intact jump graft (G) bypassing a CoA that includes a hypoplastic transverse aorta. Also note the excellent delineation of the normal RCA and LCA.* Abbreviations: *CoA, complex aortic coarctation; RCA, right coronary artery; LCA, left coronary artery.*

CLINICAL CASE 5

A 24-year-old female with Turner syndrome and Shone complex status post end-to-end coarctation repair, removal of supravalvular mitral ring, mitral commissurotomy, aortic valve replacement, and pacemaker placement presented for follow-up evaluation. Presence of an electrically active implant precluded examination with magnetic resonance imaging, prompting referral for CTA to define the postoperative anatomy and status of the aorta.

CTA showed narrowing of the transverse aorta to 9 mm just proximal to origin of the subclavian artery, a common brachiocephalic trunk arising from transverse aorta, normal dimensions of the remainder of the thoracic aorta, bileaflet tilting disk prosthetic aortic valve, pacemaker, and leads (**Fig. 10.8**). Of note, the ascending aorta was seen to lie adherent to the sternum—an important finding relevant to planning of any subsequent thoracic surgery.

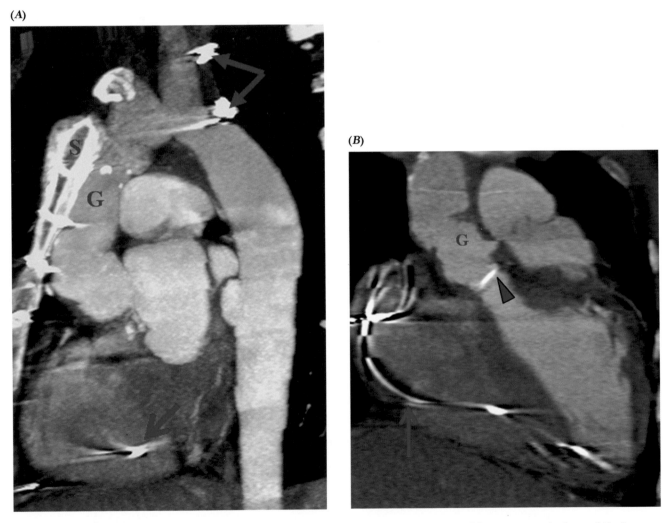

(A)

(B)

Figure 10.8 *Multiplanar reformatted (MPR) CT angiography image in an oblique sagittal plane (**A**) demonstrates the aortic repair site with mild artifact due to surgical hardware (arrows). MPR in an oblique coronal plane (**B**) shows the ascending aortic graft (G) in addition to the prosthetic aortic valve (arrowhead) and pacemaker leads (open arrows). Also note that the anterior surface of the ascending aorta/graft lies adherent to the underside of the sternum (S).*

ANEURYSM

CLINICAL CASE 6

A 52-year-old male with no past medical history presented to the emergency department for evaluation of chest pain. Physical examination was notable for bilateral arm blood pressure of 180/100 mmHg; electrocardiography demonstrated nonspecific anterior T-wave abnormality. Because of clinical suspicion of both coronary artery disease (CAD) and aortic disease, he was referred for CTA. This showed normal coronary arteries but a 5.5 cm ascending aortic aneurysm (**Fig. 10.9**).

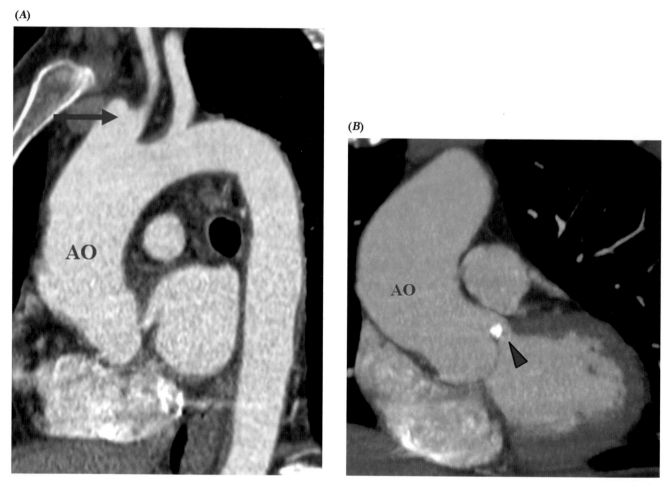

Figure 10.9 *Multiplanar reformatted CT angiography images in oblique sagittal (**A**) and coronal (**B**) planes demonstrate a 5.5 cm ascending aortic aneurysm. Also note the common brachiocephalic trunk (bovine arch anomaly, arrow) giving rise to the innominate and common carotid arteries as well mild aortic valve calcification (arrowhead).*

CLINICAL CASE 7

A 20-year-old female with aortic coarctation, prior patch aortoplasty, and subsequent transcatheter stent placement for recoarctation presented for follow-up assessment of the aortic stents. Physical examination was remarkable for a systolic ejection murmur at the suprasternal notch that radiated to the carotids bilaterally but equal blood pressures in all extremities.

Cardiac magnetic resonance examination showed bicuspid aortic valve without stenosis or insufficiency and normal left ventricular size and systolic function (EF 56%). Artifact from the aortic stents (**Fig. 10.10**) precluded adequate assessment of stent patency with magnetic resonance, prompting referral for CTA.

CTA readily demonstrated two aortic stents. The first was located between the ostia of the left common carotid and left subclavian arteries and the second had been placed just distal to the origin of the left subclavian artery (**Fig. 10.11**). Both appeared widely patent without restenosis.

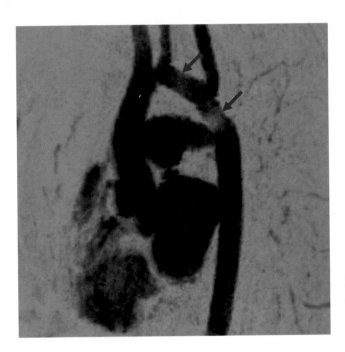

Figure 10.10 *Magnetic resonance angiogram shows stent-induced artifact in the transverse and proximal descending aorta* (arrows) *precluding adequate determination of stent patency.*

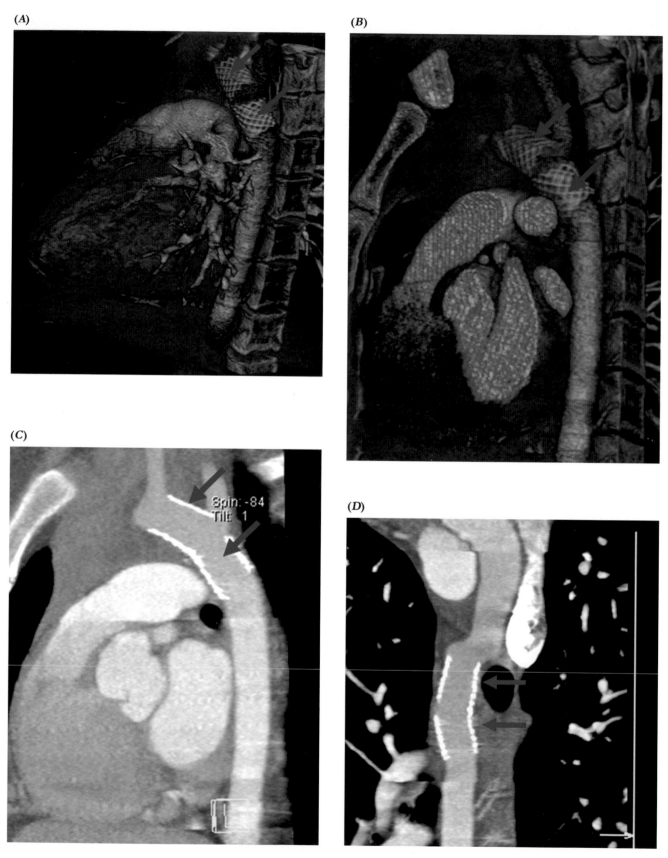

Figure 10.11 (Continued)

(E)

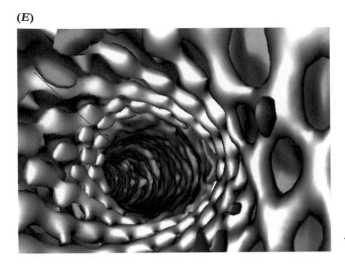

Figure 10.11 (Continued) *Volume-rendered (**A** and **B**) and multiplanar reformatted (**C** and **D**) CT angiography images demonstrate stents* (arrows) *in the transverse aorta and proximal descending thoracic aorta. An intra-aortic path (**E**, blue line) through the aortic stents further demonstrates patency (struts rendered white, vessel wall in red).*

ATHEROMATOUS DEBRIS

CLINICAL CASE 8

A 72-year-old male with hypertension, hyperlipidemia, and prior bypass surgery presented with atypical chest pain. CTA showed two of four patent grafts, normal left ventricular systolic function, and severe, diffuse aortic atheromatous debris (**Fig. 10.12**).

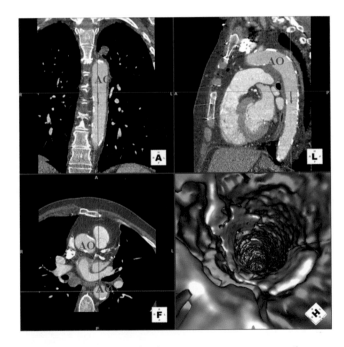

Figure 10.12 *Multiplanar reconstructions* (upper left, upper right, lower left) *and an intraluminal rendering* (lower right) *show extensive calcific atheromatous debris* (white plaques along pink vessel wall) *in the aorta (Ao).*

INTRAMURAL HEMATOMA

CLINICAL CASE 9

A 70-year-old female presented for follow-up evaluation of descending thoracic aneurysm. CTA showed aneurysmal distal descending thoracic aorta with extensive intramural hematoma: maximum aortic dimension 6.2 cm; true lumen measured 4.7 cm (**Fig. 10.13**).

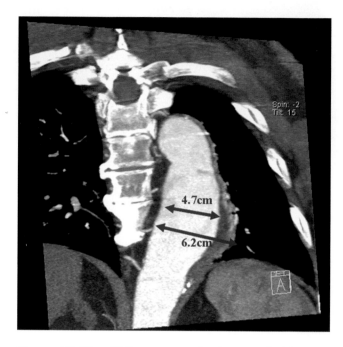

Figure 10.13 *Oblique coronal reformatted CT angiography image demonstrates intramural hematoma (*) in the mid-descending thoracic aorta.*

PENETRATING AORTIC ULCER

CLINICAL CASE 10

A 75-year-old female with hypertension and hyperlipidemia presented for evaluation of back pain. CTA demonstrated a penetrating aortic ulcer in the mid-descending thoracic aorta (**Fig. 10.14**)—the typical location for such aortic pathology. Based on stable appearance on serial imaging, the patient was managed medically.

(B)

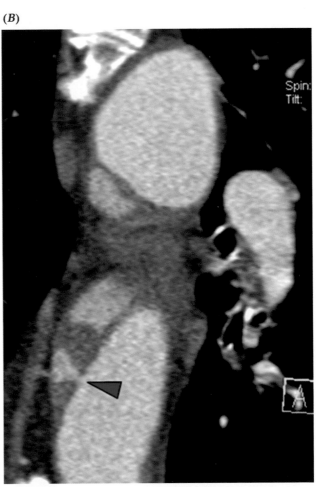

(A)

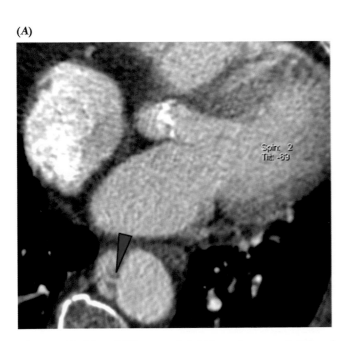

Figure 10.14   *Oblique axial (**A**) and coronal (**B**) reformatted CT angiography images demonstrate the narrow neck of a penetrating aortic ulcer in the mid-descending thoracic aorta* (arrowheads).

CLINICAL CASE 11

A 50-year-old male with hypertension, obstructive sleep apnea, hypercholesterolemia, and family history of CAD presented for evaluation of increasing dyspnea on exertion, orthopnea, and syncope. Physical examination was notable for weight of 350 pounds, a wide pulse pressure (168/56 mmHg) and grade I diastolic murmur. Cardiovascular CTA showed a ruptured sinus of Valsalva aneurysm in the right coronary sinus extending into the left ventricular outflow tract with extravasation of contrast posteriorly between the aorta and the left atrium (**Fig. 10.15**) and dilated LV with low-normal systolic function (EF 48%). Transesophageal echocardiography confirmed sinus of Valsalva aneurysm rupture with aortic valve regurgitation (**Fig. 10.16**). He then underwent resection of the aneurysm and fistulous tract and replacement of the aortic valve with a mechanical valve.

(A)

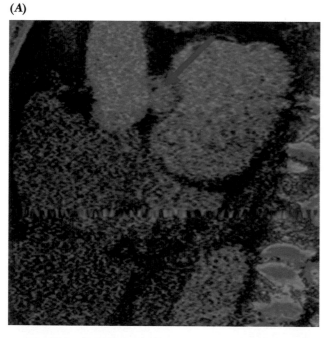

(B)

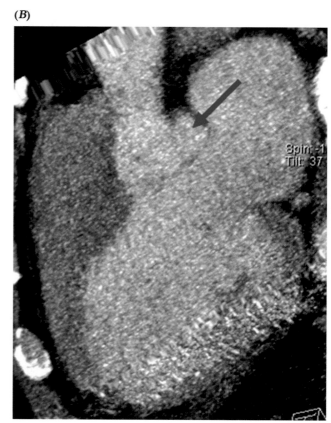

(C)

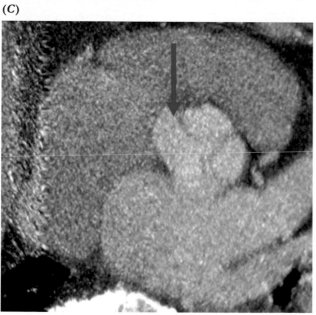

Figure 10.15 *Multiplanar reformatted CT angiography images demonstrated rupture of the noncoronary sinus of Valsalva (arrows). Image quality was severely impaired in this case by the patient's marked morbid obesity (350 pounds).*

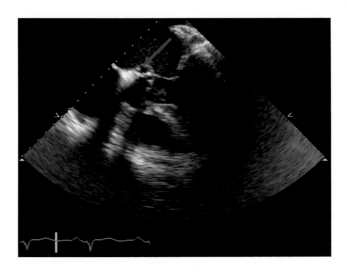

Figure 10.16 *Still frame obtained by trans-esophageal echocardiography demonstrates the ruptured sinus of Valsalva aneurysm* (arrow).

CLINICAL CASE 12

A patient presenting for routine presurgical evaluation underwent chest X ray, which revealed mediastinal widening versus possible mass adjacent to the aortic root. CTA was ordered for further diagnostic workup (**Fig. 10.17**) and demonstrated large aneurysms of the right and left aortic sinuses of Valsalva.

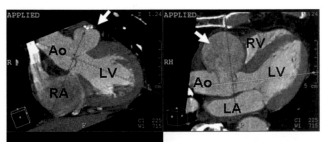

Figure 10.17 *Multiplanar reformatted CT angiography data in a patient with aneurysms of both right and left aortic sinuses of Valsalva. Frame (**A**) is an oblique right anterior projection through the thorax, demonstrating the aneurysm of the left sinus of Valsalva (arrow). Frame (**B**) is a transverse plane through the thorax/heart at the level of the aortic root, demonstrating the aneurysm of the right sinus of Valsalva (arrow). Frame (**C**) is a caudally obliqued left sagittal plane through the aortic root, demonstrating all three sinuses and the relationship of the aneurismal right and left sinuses. Note the much greater size of the right sinus aneurysm.*

CLINICAL PEARLS

- Aortic dissection can be evaluated noninvasively with CTA, avoiding potential extension with catheter-based angiography.
- CTA demonstrates the location and extent of aortic dissection, which are important factors in determining the type (e.g., A or B) of dissection as well as the need for surgical repair and/or medical therapy.
- Treatment planning in aortic dissection requires identification of the site of rupture, which can be demonstrated with review of thin-sections obtained with CTA.
- Delayed imaging (five minutes) after contrast injection allows the identification of extravasation of fluid into the false lumen of a dissection or extravascular leaks.
- CTA can provide high-resolution visualization of complex aortic anatomy due to reoperations or multiple dissections that may be difficult with other modalities such as echocardiography.
- Aortic dissection may involve the coronary arteries and great vessels; preoperative assessment of such may be demonstrated noninvasively with CTA without the risks associated with catheter-based angiography.
- Evaluation of aortic pathologies can be performed with CTA in patients with pacemakers or other metal implants that might prevent or obscure aortic imaging with other modalities.
- Aortopathy may affect the aorta and the aortic valve (e.g., bicuspid aortic valve), as well as the coronary arteries and great vessels; all of these components of aortopathy can be evaluated with CTA.
- CTA provides reproducible serial evaluation of aortic aneurysms to quantify dimensions and rate of dilatation, which has implications for timing of intervention.
- CTA allows delineation of aortic stents including patency, location, and relationship to branch vessels.
- From volumetric data, CTA images can be rendered in multiple formats including views from within the aortic lumen to assess various aspects of aortic pathologies.
- Aortic stents may produce artifact precluding intrastent assessment with modalities such as magnetic resonance; appropriate adjustment of window and level during CTA image review allows visualization of the lumen within the stent.
- Atheromatous debris in the aorta may embolize during intraoperative manipulation; CTA can provide preoperative localization of the presence and extent of aortic atherosclerosis, which may be useful, e.g., in selecting the location for cross-clamping for aortopulmonary bypass.
- Penetrating aortic ulcer and intramural hematomas are well demonstrated with CTA.
- Sinus of Valsalva aneurysm and rupture can be identified with CTA, as well as the relationship to the coronary arteries, which may be difficult with other diagnostic modalities.

Chapter 11   Cardiac masses

CLINICAL CASE 1

An 18-year-old male presented for evaluation of coronary-cameral fistula treated with transcatheter closure. Cardiac magnetic resonance imaging demonstrated a large mass in the right ventricle involving the interventricular septum that appeared bright on delayed post–gadolinium imaging (**Fig. 11.1**). CT angiography (CTA) also demonstrated the mass, as well as an intact closure device at the site of the former fistula (**Fig. 11.2**).

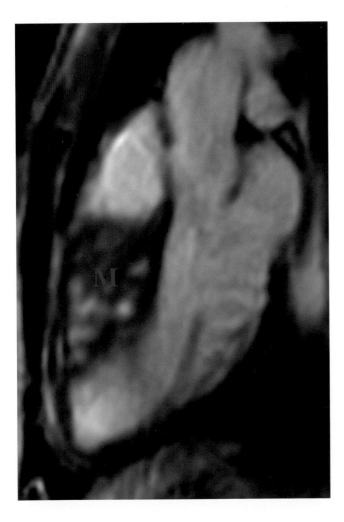

Figure 11.1 *Delayed post–gadolinium cardiac magnetic resonance image optimized for scar visualization shows an irregular mass (M) in the right ventricle. Areas of bright enhancement within the mass suggest fibrosis versus vascular components.*

(A)

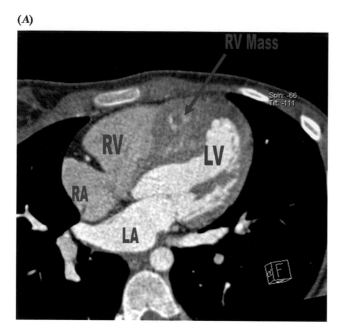

(B)

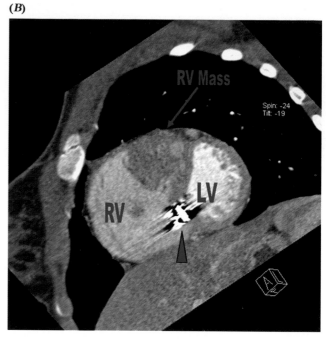

Figure 11.2 *Multiplanar CT angiography reformatted images show the right ventricle mass* (arrows) *in horizontal long axis* (**A**) *and short axis* (**B**) *planes, as well as the intact transcatheter closure device* (arrowhead).

CLINICAL CASE 2

A 36-year-old female with a history of thoracic neuroblastoma treated with radiation therapy in childhood presented for evaluation of chest pain. Coronary CTA showed normal coronary arteries but significant left atrial calcification around the left superior pulmonary vein ostium (**Fig. 11.3**).

(A)

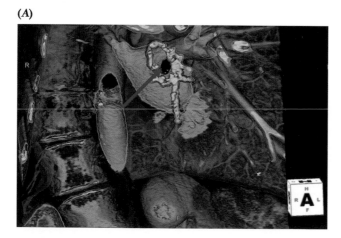

(B)

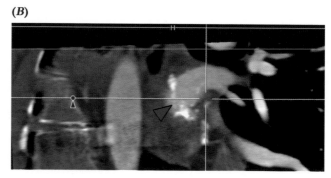

Figure 11.3 (Continued)

(C)

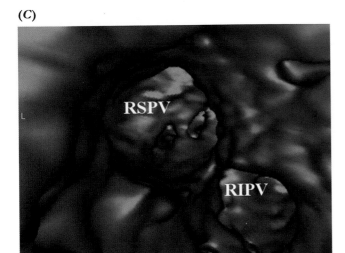

Figure 11.3 (Continued) *Volume rendering (**A**) and multiplanar reformatted (**B**) CT angiography images depict extensive calcification of the posterior left atrial wall. Note that the left inferior pulmonary vein is unobstructed* (arrow), *but the left superior pulmonary vein ostium is obscured by calcium* (arrowhead). *Volume rendering shows lack of calcification along the right side of the left atrial wall as well as the right pulmonary vein ostia (**C**).* Abbreviations: *RIPV, right inferior pulmonary vein; RSPV, right superior pulmonary vein.*

CLINICAL CASE 3

A 75-year-old male with prior percutaneous and surgical revascularization underwent echocardiography to assess left ventricular function, which was suggestive of a left ventricle (LV) apical mass (**Fig. 11.4**). Image quality was poor, even with the administration of a transpulmonic ultrasound contrast agent, prompting referral for CTA. CTA showed three patent aortocoronary bypass grafts, as well as clear demonstration of LV apical calcification and corresponding myocardial perfusion abnormality (**Fig. 11.5**).

(A)

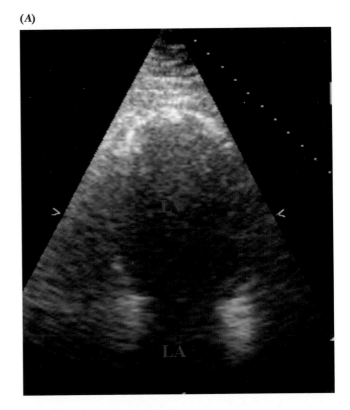

Figure 11.4 (Continued)

(B)

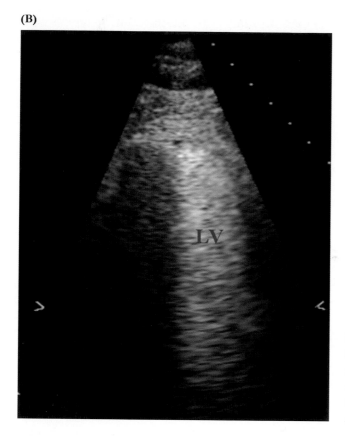

Figure 11.4 (Continued) *Surface echocardiography without (**A**) and with (**B**) administration of a transpulmonic contrast agent was suggestive of an LV apical abnormality; precise characterization was limited due to poor acoustic windows.* Abbreviations: *LA, left atrium; LV, left ventricle.*

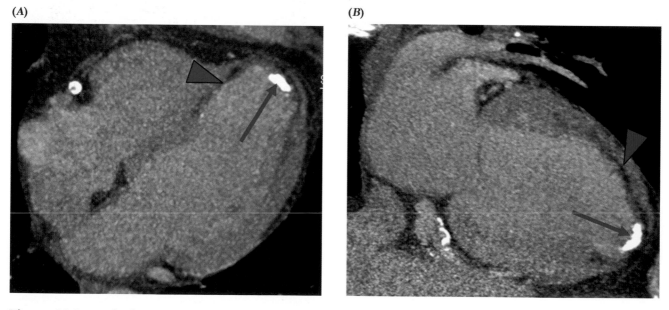

Figure 11.5 *Multiplanar reformatted CT angiography images in the horizontal long axis (**A**) and vertical long axis (**B**) planes demonstrate apical calcification (arrow) as well as marked perfusion abnormality in the left anterior descending artery distribution (arrowheads). Also note the presence of an occluded right coronary artery stent seen in cross-section (*).*

CLINICAL CASE 4

A 54-year-old patient presented with progressive dyspnea on exertion, edema, and weight loss. CTA demonstrated intracardiac histiosarcoma invading the pericardium, right atrium, right ventricle, and left atrium (**Fig. 11.6**). A malignant pleural effusion was also demonstrated in these images.

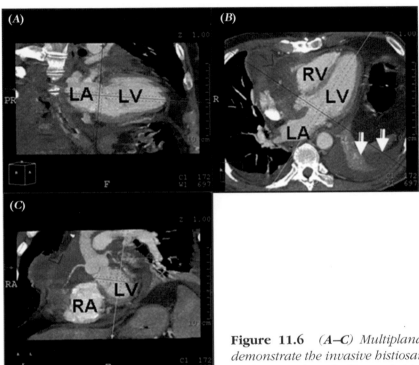

Figure 11.6 *(A–C) Multiplanar reformatted CT images of the heart demonstrate the invasive histiosarcoma* (red dashed arrows) *as well as the malignant pleural effusion* (white arrows), *visible in the left hemithorax.*

CLINICAL CASE 5

A 45-year-old male with a history of B-cell lymphoproliferative lymphoma underwent routine echocardiography for the evaluation of left ventricular function. The echocardiogram was remarkable for a mass in the left atrium; the origins and attachment of the mass were not well seen via transthoracic echocardiography, prompting cardiac CTA. The mass was well demonstrated on the CTA images (**Fig. 11.7**), including the point of attachment to the inter-atrial septum.

(A)

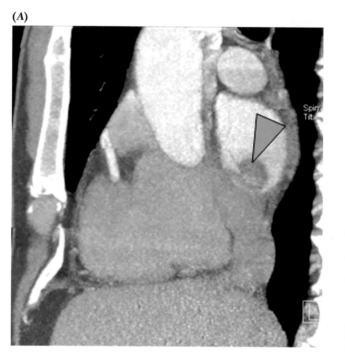

(B)

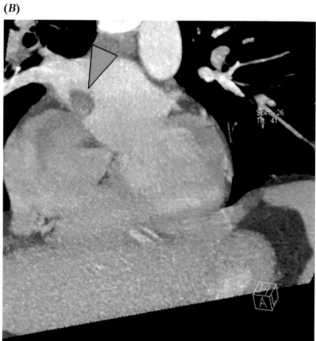

(C)

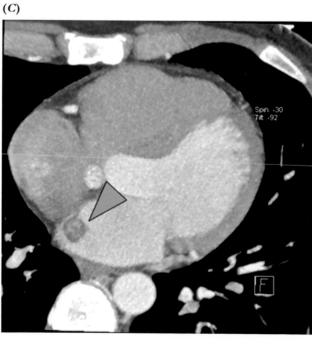

Figure 11.7 *Frame (A) demonstrates the mass in the LA from a sagittal perspective: the stalk of attachment is visible as is some contrast-enhanced stippling within the body of the mass. Frame (B) is a plane from a cranial and anterior perspective revealing the mass in relation to the LA, RA, and pulmonary vein inflow. Finally, Frame (C) reveals the mass in an axial plane demonstrating the four-chamber view of the heart, confirming the typical location and appearance of a small (1.7 × 1.4 cm) myxoma and its attachment stalk. Abbreviations: LA, left atrium; RA, right atrium.*

CLINICAL CASE 6

A patient with recurrent transient ischemic attacks presented for further evaluation. CTA demonstrated multiple intracardiac masses invading the left atrium, right atrium, and interatrial septum (**Fig. 11.8**). Examination of the mass by histopathology upon surgical removal confirmed the diagnosis of angiosarcoma.

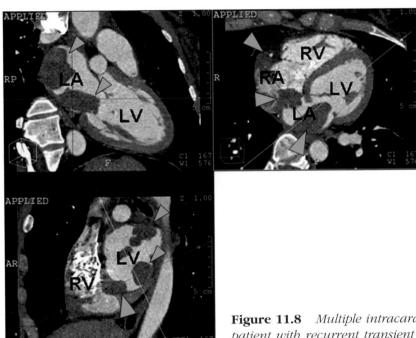

Figure 11.8 *Multiple intracardiac masses seen on CT angiography in a patient with recurrent transient ischemic attacks. The arrowheads in the frames above indicate the abnormal masses in the cardiac chambers.*

CLINICAL PEARLS

- CTA can detect intracardiac masses and delineate their size, location, and relationship to other structures.
- Cardiac masses involving calcification are particularly well visualized with CTA, such as atrial calcification due to radiation and ventricular calcification due to prior myocardial infarction.
- Left atrial calcification may obstruct the pulmonary veins; volume-rendered CTA with endoluminal visualization may be helpful in determining pulmonary venous ostial obstruction in such cases.
- CTA allows the characterization of invasiveness and border irregularities in malignant cardiac masses.
- Contrast enhancement allows determining the degree of vascularity of masses detected by CTA.
- X-ray attenuation measured in Hounsfield units identifies masses with fat, fluid, calcification, or fibrotic composition.

NORMAL CARDIAC VEINS

CLINICAL CASE 1

A 62-year-old male with atypical chest pain underwent CT angiography (CTA) for coronary evaluation. The coronary arteries were free of disease. The cardiac venous anatomy was well delineated, including the superior vena cava and coronary sinus (**Fig. 12.1**).

A "late" contrast-enhanced coronary CTA acquisition results in increased opacification of the cardiac veins. Because these venous structures often lie parallel the coronary arteries, care must be taken to distinguish coronary artery segments from cardiac vein segments (**Fig. 12.2**). This can be appreciated by tracing a questionable segment back to its origin (aorta for coronary arteries) or termination (coronary sinus for epicardial cardiac veins).

(A)

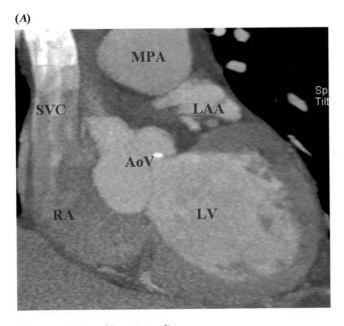

(B)

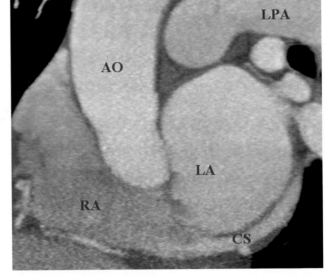

Figure 12.1   (Continued)

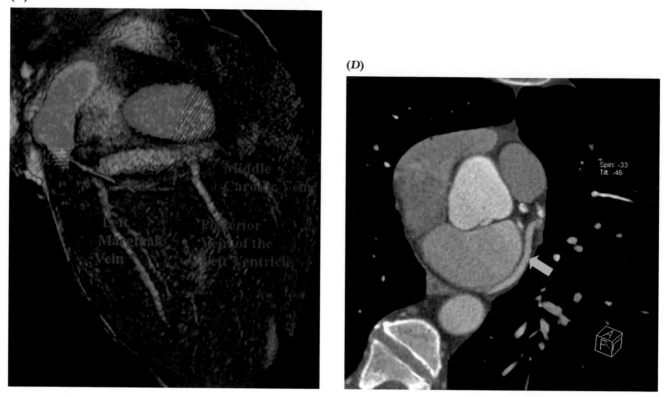

Figure 12.1 (Continued) *Multiplanar reformatted and volume-rendered CT angiography data demonstrate the normal superior vena cava (**A**) and coronary sinus anatomy (**B** and **C**). A short-axis maximum intensity projection image shows the great cardiac vein (**D**, arrow).* Abbreviations: *AO, aorta; AoV, aortic valve; LA, left atrium; LAA, left atrial appendage; LPA, left pulmonary artery; MPA, main pulmonary artery; RA, right atrium; SVC, superior vena cava; CS, coronary sinus.*

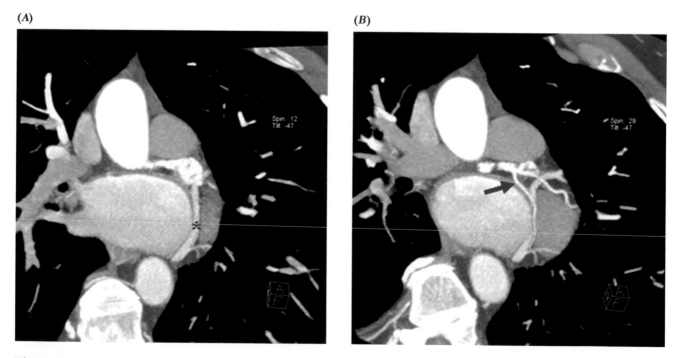

Figure 12.2 *Frame (**A**) illustrates the great cardiac vein (***), which generally lies roughly along the trajectory of the LCx for part of its course. Frame (**B**) shows a slightly different plane with both the great cardiac vein and the adjacent LCx (arrow). Note that the two vessels are opacified nearly equivalently (late timing of contrast bolus); the circumflex coronary artery can be traced back to the mainstem of the left coronary artery, whereas the great cardiac vein continues into the coronary sinus.* Abbreviation: *LCx, left circumflex coronary artery.*

ANOMOLOUS SUPERIOR VENA CAVA

CLINICAL CASE 2

A 24-year-old male with a history of repaired ventricular septal defect presented for evaluation of syncope. Further history revealed that central venous catheter placement from the left neck had been unsuccessfully attempted in the past. CTA (**Fig. 12.3**) showed a dilated coronary sinus and persistent left superior vena cava. Once the venous anatomy had been demonstrated, subsequent invasive electrophysiological testing was successfullyperformed via a right femoral venous approach.

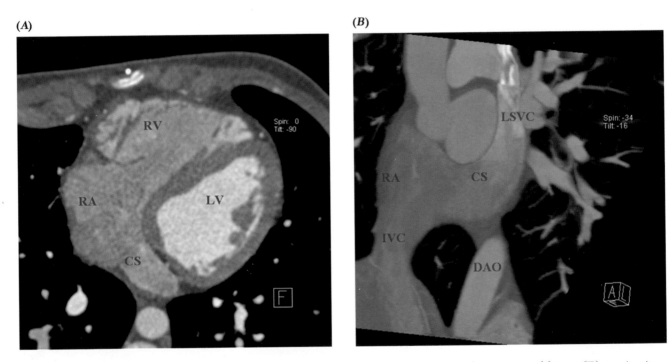

(A)

(B)

Figure 12.3 *Multiplanar reformatted CTA images in the axial (***A***) and left anterior oblique (***B***) projections demonstrate a dilated coronary sinus due to persistent LSVC. Abbreviations: LSVC, left-sided superior vena cava; CS, coronary sinus; RA, right atrium; RV, right ventricle; LV, left ventricle; IVC, inferior vena cava; DAO, descending aorta.*

PULMONARY VEINS

CLINICAL CASE 3

A 55-year-old male with risk factors for coronary artery disease underwent CTA for evaluation of shortness of breath. Coronary arteries were normal; volume rendering of the heart demonstrated normal configuration of four pulmonary veins (**Fig. 12.4**).

CLINICAL CASE 4

A 42-year-old female with severely symptomatic paroxysmal atrial fibrillation presented for evaluation of left atrial anatomy prior to radiofrequency therapy. CTA demonstrated a common left pulmonary vein (**Fig. 12.5**). The two right pulmonary veins were normal in configuration. The CT image data was directly imported into the mapping system in the electrophysiology laboratory, allowing image-guided isolation of the three pulmonary vein ostia.

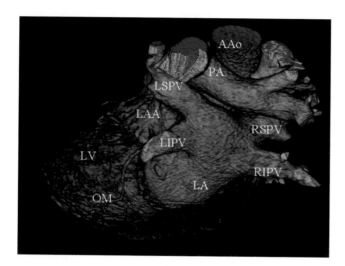

Figure 12.4 *Volume-rendered CT angiography image demonstrates normal configuration of four pulmonary veins.* Abbreviations: *AAo, ascending aorta; LA, left atrium; LAA, left atrial appendage; LIPV, left inferior pulmonary vein; LSPV, left superior pulmonary vein; LV, left ventricle; OM, obtuse marginal coronary artery; PA, pulmonary artery; RIPV, right inferior pulmonary vein; RSPV, right superior pulmonary vein.*

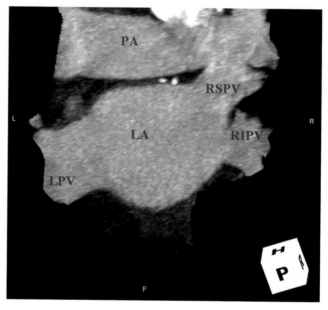

Figure 12.5 *Maximum intensity projection CT angiography image viewing the left atrium from a posterior perspective. Note the common LPV compared to two pulmonary veins on the right.* Abbreviations: *LA, left atrium; LPV, left pulmonary vein; PA, pulmonary artery; RIPV, right inferior pulmonary vein; RSPV, right superior pulmonary vein.*

CLINICAL CASE 5

A patient with chronic atrial fibrillation was referred for CTA to evaluate dyspnea following pulmonary vein isolation. CTA demonstrated complete occlusion of the right inferior pulmonary vein (**Fig. 12.6**).

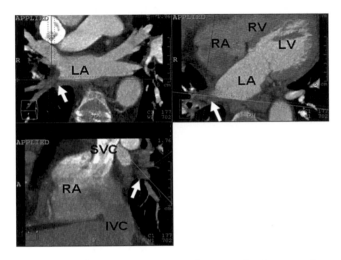

Figure 12.6 *The arrows in these multiplanar reformatted CT angiography images point to the proximal portion of the right inferior pulmonary vein, which does not contain contrast in comparison to the other pulmonary veins readily visible in the upper left panel. The lower left panel is a multiplanar reformatted image demonstrating the right inferior pulmonary vein in cross-section at the occluded site.*

CLINICAL CASE 6

A patient was referred for CTA for follow-up of pulmonary venous disease. This patient had chronic atrial fibrillation, prompting pulmonary vein isolation complicated by multiple pulmonary vein stenoses. CTA (**Fig. 12.7**) demonstrated stents in the left and right superior and left inferior veins. Mild intimal proliferation within the stent was noted in the left inferior pulmonary vein.

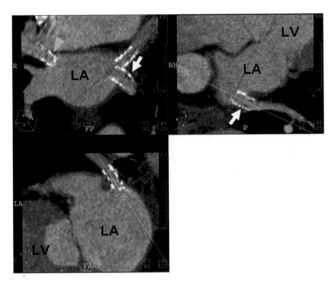

Figure 12.7 *These multiplanar reformatted CT angiography images show multiple pulmonary veins containing stents. Frame A illustrates "kissing" stents of the left inferior and superior pulmonary veins* (white arrow) *and a lone stent in the right superior pulmonary vein* (green arrowhead).

CLINICAL CASE 7

A patient with chronic atrial fibrillation who had been asymptomatic was evaluated for pulmonary vein isolation. CTA obtained postablation (**Fig. 12.8**) demonstrated moderate to severe stenosis of the left and right inferior and mild stenosis of the left superior veins. There was also associated atrial wall thickening.

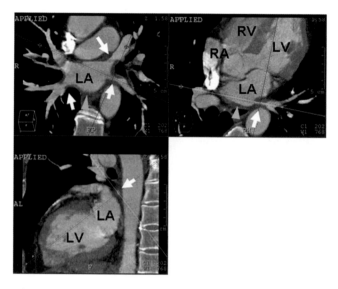

Figure 12.8 *Multiplanar reformatted CT angiography images of the left atrium and pulmonary veins in a patient with pulmonary vein stenoses. The white arrows depict the proximal portion of the pulmonary veins as they enter the left atrium. The left inferior and superior as well as the right inferior pulmonary vein exhibit some degree of stenosis. Note the associated posterior atrial wall thickening (green arrowheads).*

CLINICAL CASE 8

A patient with chronic atrial fibrillation presented for pulmonary vein isolation and underwent preprocedural CTA for the definition of vein anatomy and cardiac function. While there were no pulmonary venous anomalies, there was a marked abnormality noted in the left atrial anatomy: CTA (**Fig. 12.9**) showed prominent absence of contrast in the left atrial appendage coupled with signal intensity and contours suggestive of thrombus. The patient was on oral anticoagulation at the time.

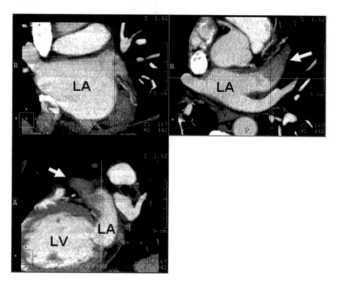

Figure 12.9 *Multiplanar reformatted images of the left atrial appendage containing thrombus in this patient with chronic atrial fibrillation (white arrow).*

CLINICAL CASE 9

A 58-year-old female underwent CTA for workup of noted absence of left pulmonary veins by catheter angiography. The patient has a history of stage III non–small cell lung cancer and had undergone chemotherapy and radiation therapy to her chest 4.5 years prior to her presentation. She presented to the emergency room with congestive heart failure and was found to have severely elevated pulmonary pressures by right heart catheterization. Further imaging and catheterization revealed absence of both left-sided pulmonary veins and the left pulmonary artery. The residual stub of the left pulmonary veins is also illustrated (**Fig. 12.10**).

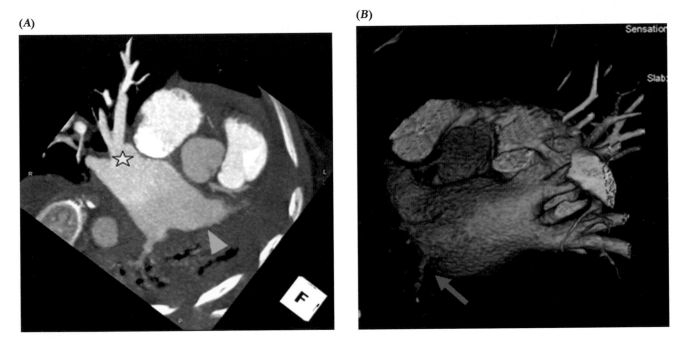

(A)

(B)

Figure 12.10   *Frame (A) is a maximum intensity projection CT angiography image through the LA depicting the origin of the left* (red arrow) *and right pulmonary veins (star), as well as the proximal conduit into the LA appendage* (green arrowhead). *Note the left pulmonary vein is obliterated. The right pulmonary veins (including a right middle pulmonary vein—distinct ostium not well demonstrated in this plane) appear normal. Frame (B) is the volume-rendered posterior view of the LA, once again illustrating the atretic left pulmonary vein* (red arrow) *and the intact right pulmonary veins.* Abbreviation: *LA, left atrium.*

CLINICAL PEARLS

- Cardiac venous anatomy can be well defined with CTA.
- To visualize right heart venous structures such as the coronary sinus, acquisition timing to insure appearance of contrast in the right heart may be helpful compared to routine coronary CTA protocols that optimize appearance of contrast in the left heart and aorta.
- Venous anomalies such as persistent left superior vena cava or pulmonary vein anomalies may have important implications when performing transvenous diagnostic or therapeutic procedures. These anomalies can be recognized prior to such procedures with CTA, potentially minimizing in-lab complications.
- CTA may help delineate coronary sinus anatomy prior to placement of transvenous leads for biventricular pacing that may be helpful for patients with cardiac dyssynchrony.
- Prior to catheter ablation procedures for atrial fibrillation, CTA provides a detailed assessment of left atrial and pulmonary vein anatomy.
- After catheter ablation procedures, CTA can help identify pulmonary vein stenosis, including assessment of severity and progression.

Chapter 13   Peripheral artery disease

CAROTID ARTERIES

CLINICAL CASE 1

A 70-year-old female with coronary artery disease, hypertension, and hyperlipidemia presented for evaluation of progressive carotid artery disease by ultrasonography.

Physical examination was notable for a right-sided carotid bruit. Doppler ultrasound suggested right carotid artery stenosis >70%, with a high peak systolic velocity and an elevated end-diastolic velocity. CT angiography (CTA) showed comparable high-grade luminal narrowing of the right internal carotid artery (**Fig. 13.1**). She subsequently underwent successful right carotid endarterectomy (**Fig. 13.2**).

(A)

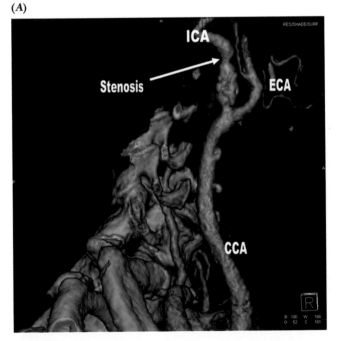

(B)

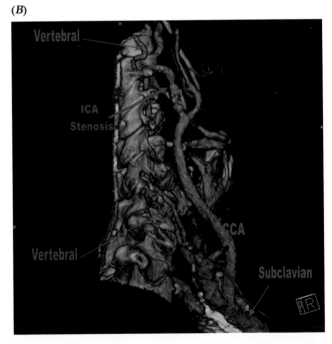

Figure 13.1 *Volume-rendered CT angiography images demonstrate a complex stenosis in the proximal portion of the right internal carotid artery.*

(A)

(B)

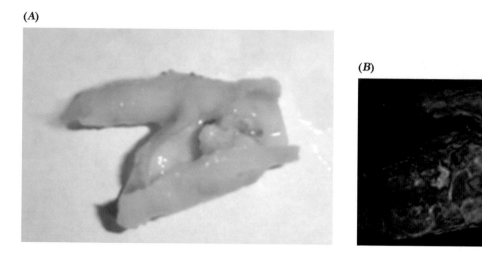

Figure 13.2   *Photograph of the explanted plaque obtained at the time of carotid endarterectomy (**A**) and corresponding magnetic resonance image of the specimen (**B**).*

CLINICAL CASE 2

A 61-year-old male with hypertension and diabetes presented for routine health maintenance. A right carotid bruit was appreciated on physical examination, prompting referral for CTA. CTA showed high-grade right internal carotid artery stenosis (**Fig. 13.3**). He also underwent magnetic resonance angiography that showed similar high-grade stenosis (**Fig. 13.4**). He subsequently underwent right carotid endarterectomy; magnetic resonance imaging of the explanted plaque confirmed the in vivo findings (**Fig. 13.5**).

(A)

(B)

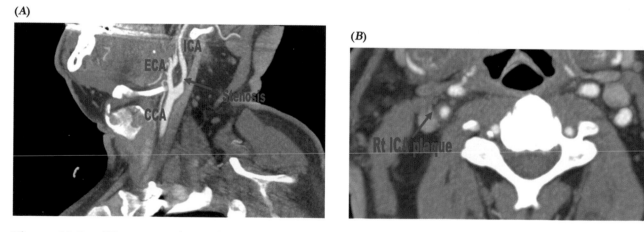

Figure 13.3   *CT angiography multiplanar reformatted images along the length of the right internal carotid artery (**A**) as well as in cross-section show both the high-grade stenosis (**A**, arrow) and the noncalcified plaque producing the stenosis (**B**, arrow).*

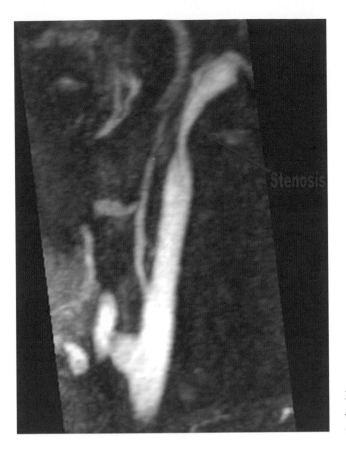

Figure 13.4 *Magnetic resonance angiogram in the same individual shows the stenosis of the right internal carotid artery* (arrow).

(A)

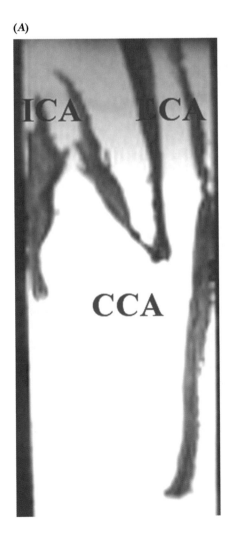

(B)

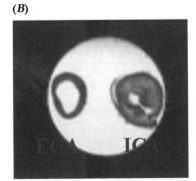

Figure 13.5 *Magnetic resonance imaging of the explanted plaque obtained at the time of carotid endarterectomy confirms high-grade stenosis in the right internal carotid artery both along its long axis (A) and in cross-section (B).* Abbreviations: *CCA, common carotid artery; ECA, external carotid artery; ICA, internal carotid artery.*

RENAL ARTERIES

CLINICAL CASE 3

A 65-year-old female with poorly controlled hypertension presented for noninvasive assessment of the renal arteries. Physical examination was notable for an abdominal bruit. CT angiography (**Fig. 13.6**) showed high-grade left renal artery stenosis and diffuse aortic atherosclerosis without obstruction extending into the common iliac arteries. She subsequently underwent left renal artery balloon angioplasty and stent implantation from the right femoral approach.

(B)

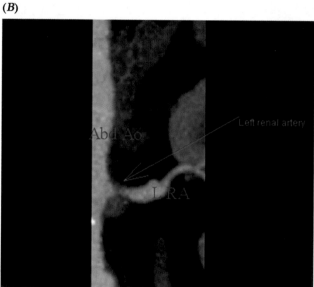

(A)

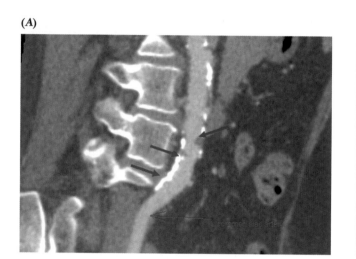

Figure 13.6 *CT angiography images demonstrating diffuse aortoiliac atherosclerosis (**A***, arrows) and high-grade stenosis in the left renal artery (**B**). Abbreviations: Abd Ao, abdominal aorta; LRA, left renal artery.*

CLINICAL CASE 4

An 82-year-old female with a history of right renal artery stenosis status post stent placement presented for evaluation of episodic dizziness and blood pressure fluctuations. CTA was ordered as part of the workup to assess for patency of the previously placed stent as well as progression of renal artery occlusive disease. Multiplanar reformatted (MPR), maximum intensity projection, and volume-rendered images (**Fig. 13.7**) nicely demonstrated patency of the right renal artery stent and moderate plaque in the left renal artery.

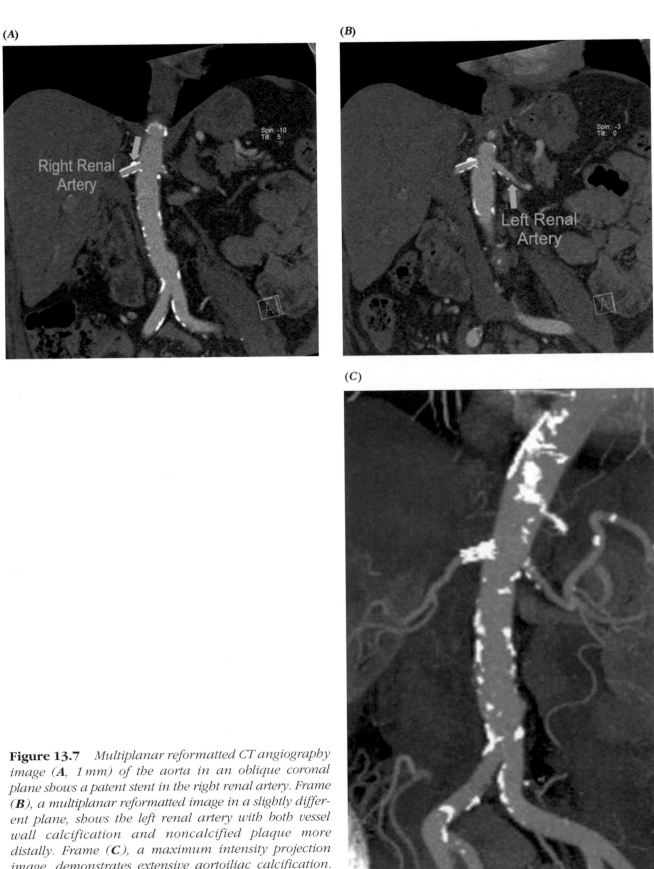

Figure 13.7 *Multiplanar reformatted CT angiography image (**A**, 1 mm) of the aorta in an oblique coronal plane shows a patent stent in the right renal artery. Frame (**B**), a multiplanar reformatted image in a slightly different plane, shows the left renal artery with both vessel wall calcification and noncalcified plaque more distally. Frame (**C**), a maximum intensity projection image, demonstrates extensive aortoiliac calcification. Note that when rendered in this fashion, the stent lumen cannot be appreciated due to overlapping sections.*

SUBCLAVIAN STENOSIS

CLINICAL CASE 5

A 72-year-old female with coronary artery disease and prior bypass surgery including left internal mammary artery (LIMA) to the left anterior descending coronary artery subsequently developed subclavian artery stenosis that was treated with percutaneous stent placement complicated by stroke. Routine stress testing suggested anterior perfusion abnormality versus breast attenuation artifact. Rather than undergo repeat invasive angiography, the patient was referred for CTA. This demonstrated patency of the LIMA and subclavian artery stent with significant calcific plaque at the origin of the subclavian artery, as well as moderate stenosis distal to the stent (**Fig. 13.8**). Because the patient was asymptomatic, she elected to pursue more aggressive medical management.

(A)

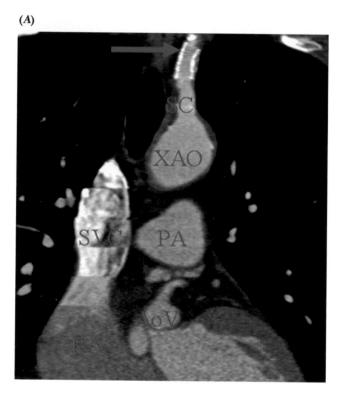

(B)

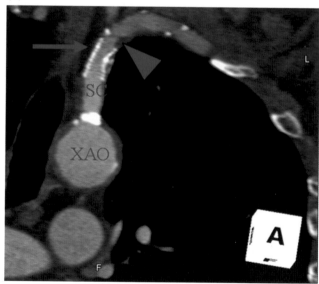

Figure 13.8   (Continued)

(C)

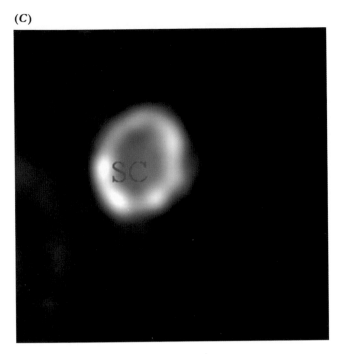

(D)

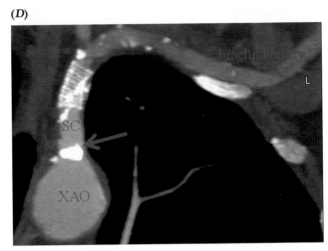

Figure 13.8 (Continued) *Multiplanar reformatted images (**A–C**) and maximum intensity projection CT angiography image (**D**) show a patent proximal SC stent* (arrow) *lengthwise and in cross-section with moderate stenosis distal to the stent* (arrowhead), *as well as diffuse mild plaque in the mid and distal SC (**D**). Note the severe calcification (**D**, open arrow) at the origin of the SC from the transverse aorta (XAO).* Abbreviations: *AoV, aortic valve; RA, right atrium; SC, subclavian artery; SVC, superior vena cava.*

AORTOILIAC DISEASE

CLINICAL CASE 6

An 85-year-old male with hypertension and a remote smoking history had undergone prior transcatheter placement of an aortoiliac bifurcated stent graft device to treat an infrarenal abdominal aortic aneurysm. He was referred for CTA for post–endovascular therapy follow-up. The device was well visualized (**Fig. 13.9**), with no endoleaks. Proximal and distal attachments were well seated.

(A)

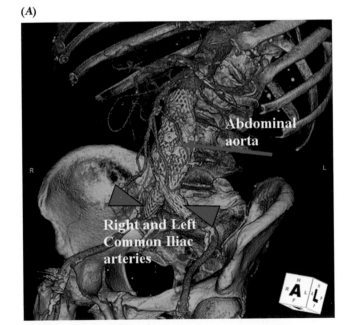

Figure 13.9 (Continued)

(B)

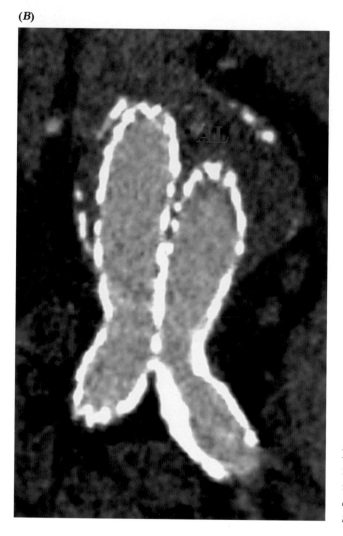

Figure 13.9 (Continued) *CT angiography volume-rendered (A) and coronal multiplanar reformatted (B) images show an intact aortoiliac bifurcating stent graft device. Note the absence of contrast in the excluded portion of the AL in (B).* Abbreviation: *AL, aneurysm lumen.*

CLINICAL CASE 7

The images in **Figures 13.10** to **13.12** are from a patient referred for peripheral CTA to assess aortobifemoral graft status. The images illustrate that the graft is patent, with good contrast opacification of the femoral arteries and the lower extremity arteries showing at least two vessel below-knee runoff bilaterally. As with coronary CTA imaging, the key to obtaining good quality peripheral CTA images is modulation of the contrast delivery and scan time. A steady, slow contrast injection delivery rate (usually using bolus tracking techniques) can result in optimal vessel opacification equal or superior to invasive x-ray angiography with the additional advantages of multiplanar interrogation of the data and capabilities such as three-dimensional rendering. While volumetric visualizations provide an appealing format for overall assessment, it is crucial to examine thin-section MPR images (**Fig. 13.11**), preferably in the plane axial to the length of the vessel and at least one orthogonal plane, to formulate a diagnosis of disease in that vessel. Three-dimensional reformatted images are prone to human and technical manipulation, whereas the thin-section images in the axial or MPR format contain the unmanipulated data limited only by adequacy of acquisition technique.

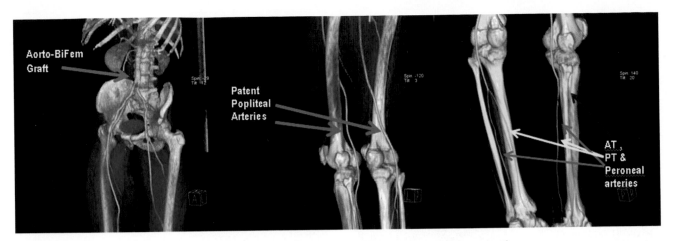

Figure 13.10 *The three-dimensional volume-rendered CT angiography data provides an overview of the aortoiliac and lower leg arteries with anatomic landmarks nicely demonstrated by inclusion of the bony structures. Abbreviations: AT, anterior tibial artery; PT, posterior tibial artery.*

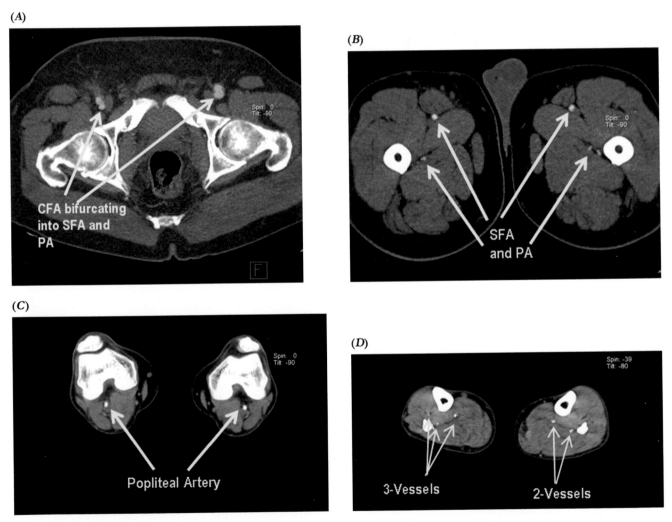

Figure 13.11 *Multiplanar reconstructed images of different anatomic levels of the lower extremity arterial tree. Frame (**A**) is a planar section through the pelvis at the level of the bifurcation of the CFA into the superficial femoral and profunda femoris. Frame (**B**) is an axial plane through the upper thighs, depicting the SFA and the PA in cross-section at that level. Frame (**C**) is an axial section of the legs at the level of the patellae, illustrating the patent popliteal artery in its course behind the knee. Frame (**D**) shows the three-vessel runoff in the right lower extremity and the two vessel runoff in the left lower extremity mid-way between the knees and ankles. Abbreviations: CFA, common femoral artery; PA, profunda artery; SFA, superficial femoral artery.*

(A)

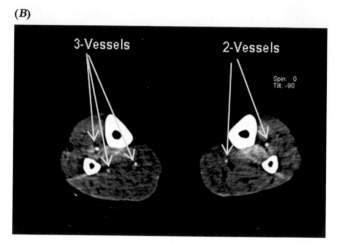

Figure 13.12 *This is a peripheral CT angiogram illustrating a "thin-slab" maximum intensity projection (MIP) which is an optional method for reconstructing three-dimensional (3-D) CT angiography data. Frame (**A**): the image shown is in grayscale with volume-rendered contrast-opacified vasculature. This image enables an overall 3-D assessment of the entire vasculature of the legs. Most software packages allow this type of reconstruction from submillimeter to multimillimeter sections of the thin-slice axial data. This particular package allows for "bone removal" as well ("negative" contrast within the soft tissue density of the legs). Once the survey has allowed for identification of any diseased segments, those segments can be examined more carefully as axial sections (Frame **B**). Frame (**B**) demonstrates the three vessels seen in the right lower extremity and the two vessels seen in the left lower extremity of the MIP in Frame (**A**).*

CLINICAL PEARLS

- Vascular stent evaluation requires CTA data review in multiple image planes, including along the length of the stent as well as in cross-section. Curved MPR images may be useful in demonstrating nonlinear stented segments.

- Carotid artery disease can be assessed with CTA, including location of stenoses, type of plaque, and measurement of vessel lumen and vessel wall diameters.

- After percutaneous stent placement, restenosis may develop within the stent as well as just proximally or just distally to the stent. Careful review of all vessel segments allows accurate recognition of postintervention stenoses.

- Subclavian stenosis is important to identify in patients undergoing bypass graft surgery using the internal mammary artery as a conduit. Postoperative assessment in such patients should also include imaging of the subclavian artery; both LIMA and the subclavian artery may be imaged simultaneously with CTA.

- CTA has become the preferred modality for long-term follow-up of endovascular repairs, because it allows noninvasive detection of device patency, migration, and leaks.

Chapter 14   Congenital heart disease

ACYANOTIC LESIONS

VENTRICULAR SEPTAL DEFECT

Clinical Case 1

A 34-year-old female with a long-standing harsh systolic murmur presented for evaluation of chest pain. Coronary CT angiography (CTA) showed a perimembranous (conoventricular) ventricular septal defect (VSD), normal systolic function, and no disease in the coronary arteries (**Fig. 14.1**).

(A)

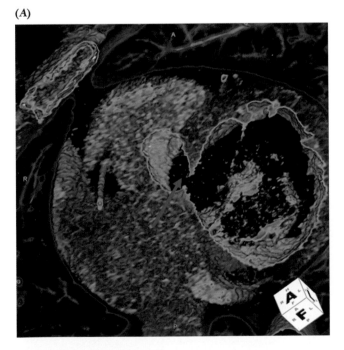

(B)

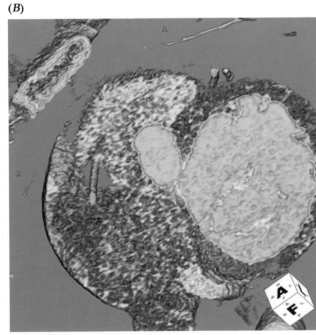

Figure 14.1 (Continued)

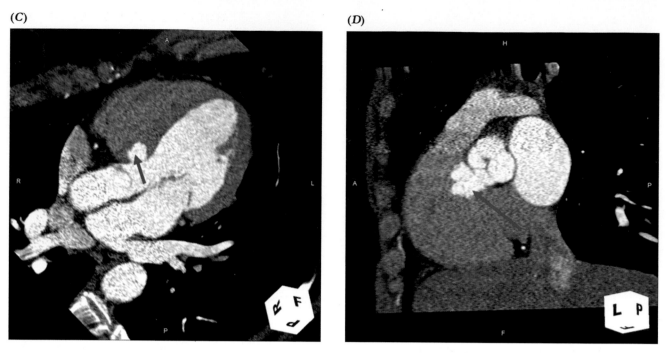

Figure 14.1 (Continued) (**A**) Volume rendering at the basal short axis level demonstrates a ventricular septal defect (arrow). (**B**) Volume rendering at same level using inverted grey scale. (**C**) Maximum intensity projection image in a long axis plane shows the ventricular septal defect (arrow). (**D**) An oblique sagittal maximum intensity projection image demonstrating the perimembranous ventricular septal defect (arrow).

Clinical Case 2

A 30-year-old male with hypertension and a strong family history of premature coronary artery disease presented for evaluation of atypical chest pain.

Coronary CTA showed isolated plaque disease of the coronary arteries and normal systolic function of the left ventricle (LV). A healed muscular VSD was identified (**Fig. 14.2**).

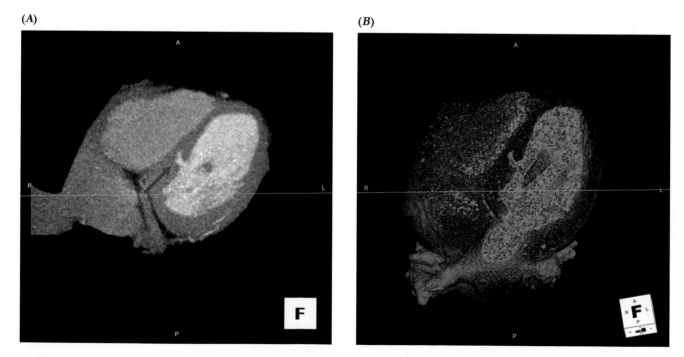

Figure 14.2 (**A**) Maximum intensity projection image demonstrates a healed muscular ventricular septal defect (arrow). (**B**) Volume rendered image again demonstrates the muscular ventricular septal defect. Note that it no longer connects with the right ventricle, indicating spontaneous closure.

COARCTATION OF THE AORTA

Clinical Case 3

A 36-year-old male with a history of bicuspid aortic valve and coarctation of the aorta, who had undergone an end-to-end anastomosis with resection of the coarctation segment, presented for evaluation of systolic hypertension despite aggressive antihypertensive therapy. Previously this patient had also required balloon aortoplasty for recurrent coarctation. A CT was obtained to assess the aorta and coronary arteries (**Figs. 14.3–14.5**).

(A)

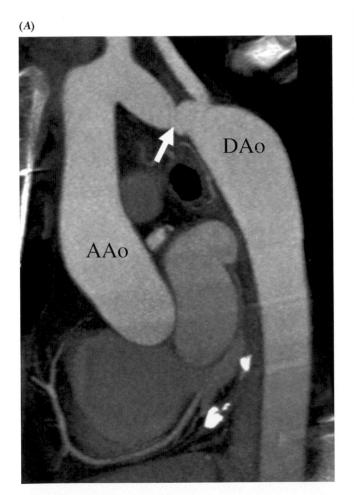

(B)

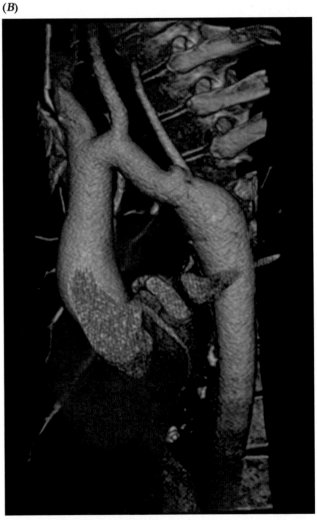

Figure 14.3 *An oblique sagittal view (**A**) and volume rendered three-dimensional reconstruction (**B**) identify the complex appearance of the aortic arch. The ascending aorta (AAo) is mildly dilated. The transverse arch is diffusely hypoplastic that tapers at the previous site of coarctation repair (white arrow) with post-stenotic dilatation of the proximal descending aorta (DAo). Abbreviations: AAo, ascending aorta; DAo, descending aorta.*

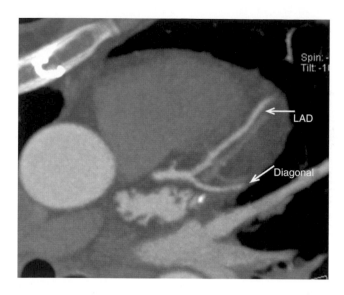

Figure 14.4 *An oblique axial view demonstrates the normal anatomy of the left anterior descending (LAD) coronary artery and a diagonal branch.*

(B)

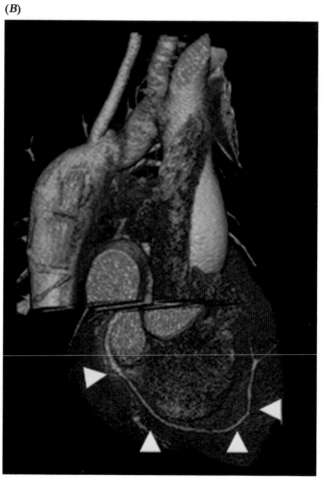

(A)

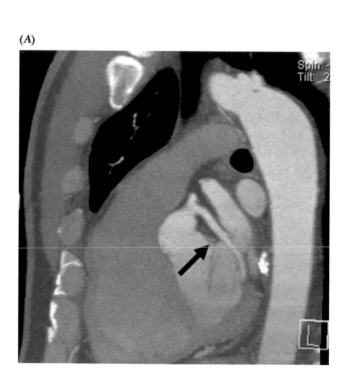

Figure 14.5 *The right coronary artery was never identified. However, the proximal circumflex artery* (black arrow) *is seen on the oblique sagittal view* (**A**), *which continues along the anterior atrioventricular groove in the distribution of the right coronary artery* (yellow arrowheads) *seen on the volume rendered three-dimensional reconstruction* (**B**).

Clinical Case 4

A 37-year-old male with bicuspid aortic valve and coarctation of the aorta underwent an end-to-end anastomosis and later presented for a routine follow-up evaluation (**Fig. 14.6–14.8**).

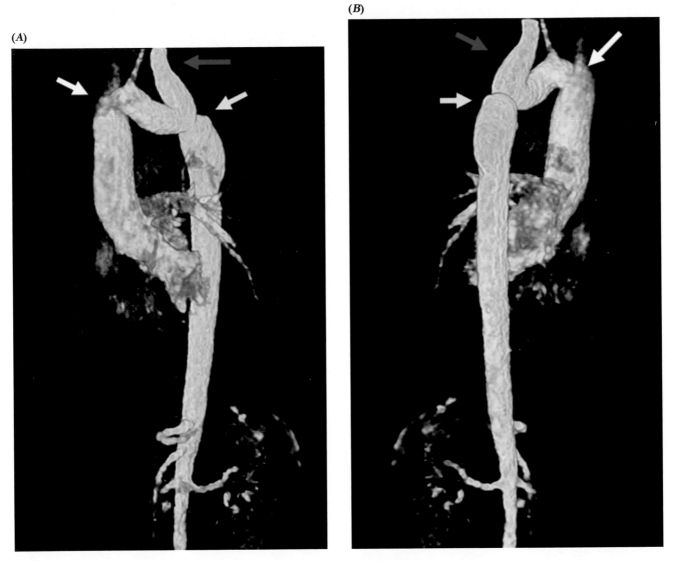

Figure 14.6 *Three-dimensional magnetic reconstruction in the anterior (**A**) and posterior (**B**) projections demonstrate the complex anatomy of the aorta. There appears to be a fold in the distal ascending aorta* (white arrow), *dilatation of the left subclavian artery* (red arrow), *and an area of recoarctation* (yellow arrow).

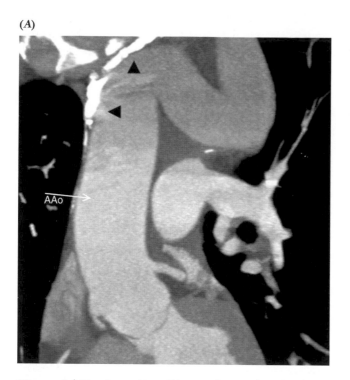

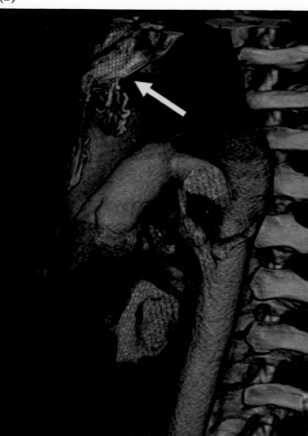

Figure 14.7 *A cardiac CT was obtained to further assess the fold in the distal ascending aorta. Areas of calcification* (arrowheads) *can be identified in this oblique coronal view* (**A**). *A volume rendered three-dimensional reconstruction* (**B**) *demonstrates that this portion of the aorta is adherent to the sternum* (arrow) *with small collateral vessels noted in this vicinity. This information is of critical importance in order to plan transcatheter relief of any residual coarctation.*

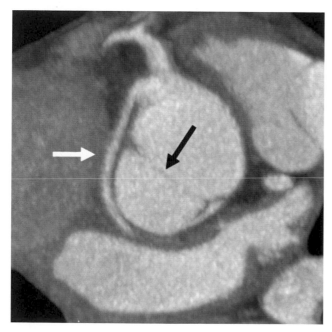

Figure 14.8 *An oblique axial view demonstrates a bicuspid aortic valve* (black arrow) *and anomalous origin of left circumflex* (white arrow) *that arises from a distinct ostia coursing posterior to the aorta without evidence of coronary artery atherosclerosis.*

Clinical Case 5

A 28-year-old male with a history of coarctation of the aorta initially underwent an end-to-end anastomosis, but later required a patch aortoplasty and finally placement of jump graft to address severe recoarctation. A CT was obtained to evaluate the anatomy of the entire aortic arch and the jump graft (**Fig. 14.9**).

(B)

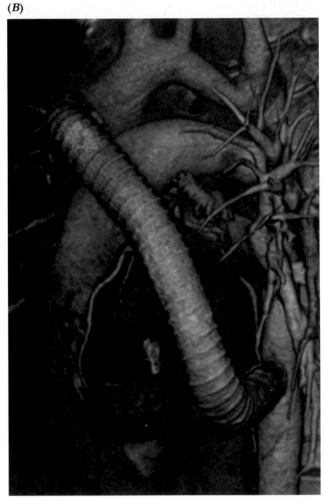

(A)

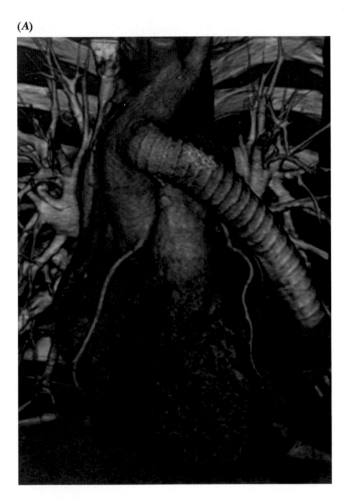

Figure 14.9 (Continued)

(C)

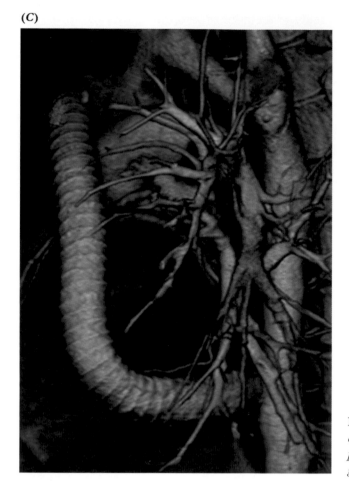

Figure 14.9 (Continued) *Volume rendered three-dimensional reconstructions exquisitely delineate the proximal (**A**), mid (**B**), and distal (**C**) aspects of the jump graft as well as the anatomy of the native aortic arch.*

SUPRAVALVULAR AORTIC STENOSIS

Clinical Case 6

A 29-year-old obese male with William's syndrome associated with supravalvular aortic stenosis and hypertension underwent a cardiac CT to evaluate symptoms of chest pain (**Figs. 14.10** and **14.11**).

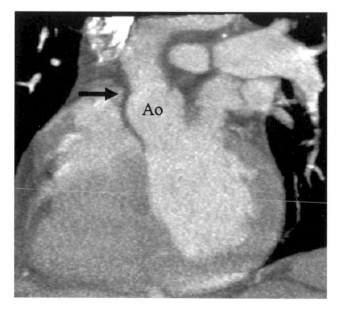

Figure 14.10 *An oblique coronal view demonstrates the "hourglass" appearance of the Ao in patients with supravalvular aortic stenosis (arrow). Abbreviation: Ao, ascending aorta.*

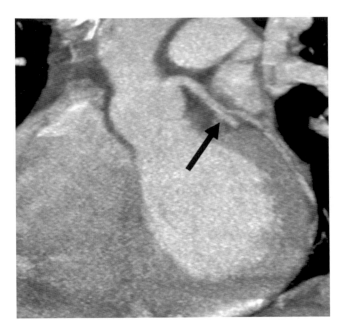

Figure 14.11   *An oblique coronal view delineates the anatomy of the proximal left anterior descending coronary artery* (arrow) *without evidence of plaque.*

PULMONARY VALVE STENOSIS

Clinical Case 7

A 48-year-old female with history of Noonan's syndrome and complex subpulmonic and pulmonary valve stenosis who had previously undergone placement of a right ventricle-to-pulmonary artery (RV–PA) conduit presented for evaluation of shortness of breath. A significant gradient along the conduit had been identified with transthoracic echocardiography. Prior to conduit revision, a cardiac CT was performed to delineate the anatomy of her coronary arteries, which had been reported as "abnormal" (**Fig. 14.12**).

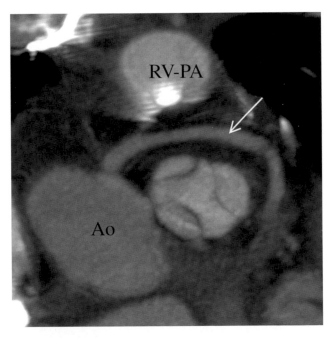

Figure 14.12   *An oblique axial view demonstrated a single coronary from the right cusp of the aortic valve* (arrow). *Importantly, the left main coursed between the native right ventricular outflow tract and the RV–PA conduit which provides important information prior to additional surgical revisions of the conduit. The pulmonary valve leaflets appear thickened and dysplastic—features commonly seen in Noonan's patients.*

ATRIAL SEPTAL DEFECT AND VSD

Clinical Case 8

A 33-year-old male with history of atrial septal defect (ASD) and VSDs initially underwent a palliative repair with a PA band, which was later followed by complete repair with take-down of the band. Subsequently, this patient was lost to follow-up and then returned with significant shortness of breath. A cardiac magnetic resonance imaging (MRI) study identified bilateral proximal PA stenosis requiring transcatheter intervention with placement of stents in both the proximal left and the right pulmonary arteries. A follow-up cardiac CT was performed to assess stent patency (**Figs. 14.13** and **14.14**).

(A)

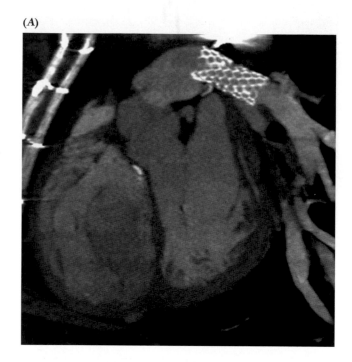

(B)

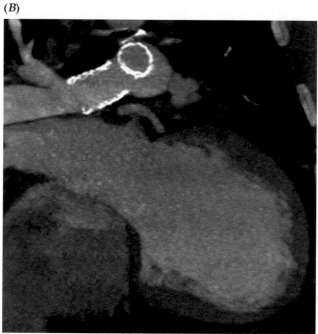

Figure 14.13 *An oblique coronal view demonstrates the exterior surface of the stent deployed in the left pulmonary artery with flow in the distal pulmonary arteries suggesting patency (**A**). Another oblique coronal view (**B**) demonstrates patency of the right pulmonary artery stent longitudinally and patency of the left pulmonary artery stent from a cross-sectional view.*

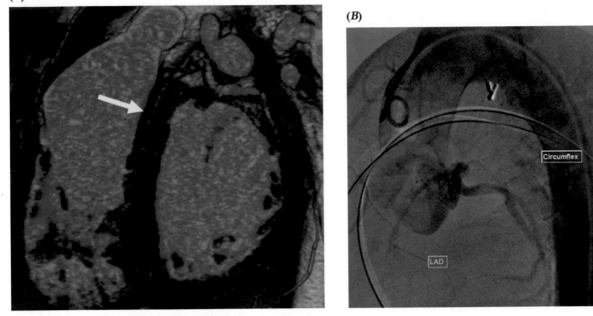

Figure 14.14 *A volume rendered three-dimensional reconstruction (**A**) also identified a hypoplastic appearance of the left anterior descending (LAD) coronary artery (arrow). The cardiac catheterization (**B**) was retrospectively reviewed to confirm these findings: aortic root angiography demonstrates the diffusely hypoplastic LAD in comparison to the normal caliber of the circumflex artery.*

VSD AND PULMONAY VALVE STENOSIS

Clinical Case 9

A 26-year-old female with a history of VSD and pulmonary stenosis having undergone patch closure of the VSD and pulmonary valvectomy and "reportedly" anomalous coronaries underwent a cardiac CT to assess her RV size and function and to assess the coronaries and anatomy of the right ventricular outflow tract (**Figs. 14.15–14.18**).

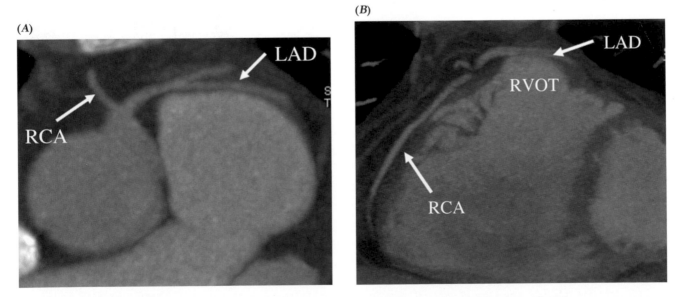

Figure 14.15 *An oblique axial view (**A**) demonstrates the left anterior descending (LAD) coronary artery arising from the right coronary artery (RCA). The oblique coronal view (**B**) demonstrates that the LAD traverses anterior to the right ventricular outflow tract (RVOT).*

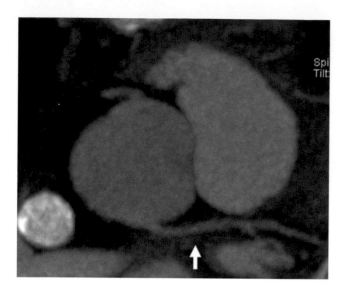

Figure 14.16 *An oblique axial view demonstrates the circumflex coronary artery arising from left coronary cusp of the aortic valve.*

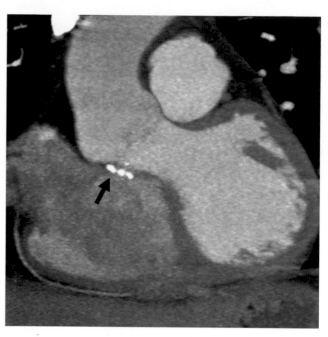

Figure 14.17 *Patch closure of the ventricular septal defect can be identified by the focal area of calcification within the interventricular septum* (arrow) *in this oblique coronal view.*

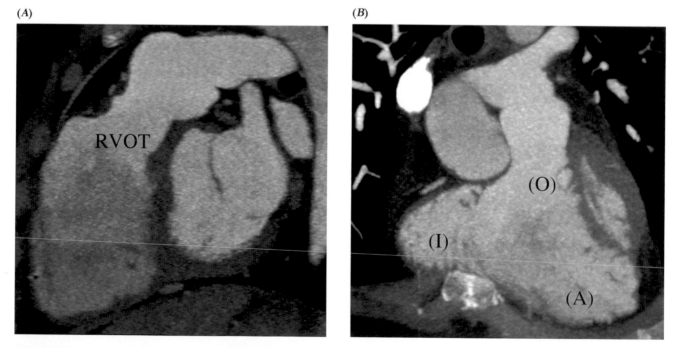

Figure 14.18 *The anatomy of the right ventricular outflow tract (RVOT) is accurately delineated in the oblique sagittal view (**A**). The oblique coronal view (**B**) demonstrates the tripartite appearance of the right ventricle including the inlet (I), apical (A), and outflow (O) segments.*

ATRIOVENTRICULAR SEPTAL DEFECT

Clinical Case 10

A 53-year-old female with a history of an atrioventricular septal defect underwent complete repair and was later found to have right PA stenosis requiring transcatheter relief with implantation of a stent, hypertension, and diabetes mellitus type II presented with increasing dyspnea (at rest and with exertion), orthopnea, and lower extremity edema. A cardiac CT was obtained to evaluate stent patency and right ventricular function and assess the coronary arterial tree (**Figs. 14.19** and **14.20**).

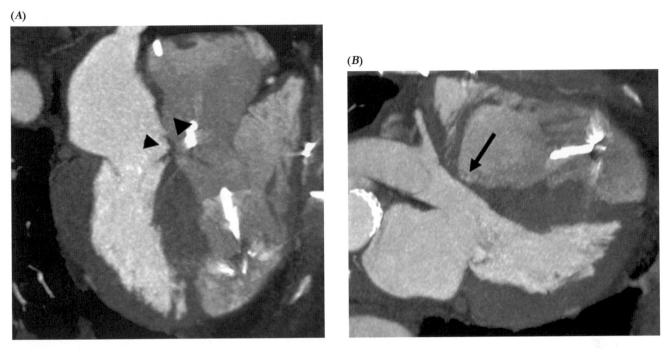

Figure 14.19 *The classic features of a repaired atrioventricular septal defect are seen, including the left and right atrioventricular valves* (arrowheads) *along the same plane* (**A**) *and the "goose-neck" deformity* (arrow) *of the left-ventricular outflow tract* (**B**).

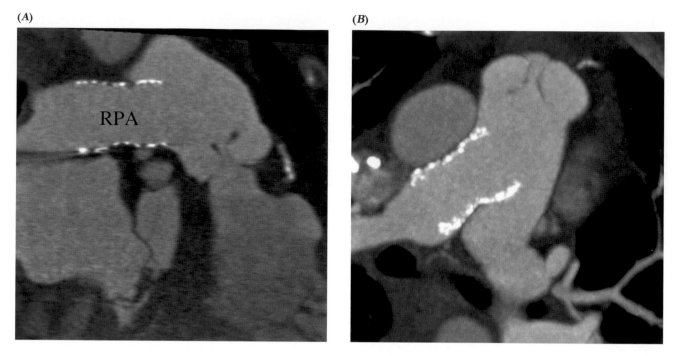

Figure 14.20 *Oblique coronal (**A**) and axial (**B**) views demonstrate the patency of the right pulmonary artery (RPA) stent. In addition, the pulmonary valve leaflets appear slightly thickened and dysplastic.*

CYANOTIC LESIONS

TETRALOGY OF FALLOT

Clinical Case 11

A 69-year-old male with tetralogy of Fallot underwent initial palliative repair with a classic left-sided Blalock–Taussig shunt at the age of 10 and ultimately a complete repair at age 46 in 1982. He also has a past medical history significant for hypertension, hyperlipidemia, tobacco addiction, type II diabetes mellitus, and atherosclerotic coronary artery disease and has required percutaneous coronary intervention on the right coronary artery (RCA). He presented with worsening shortness of breath and right ventricular failure. A cardiac CT was obtained to assess the patency of the RCA stent and evaluate RV function (**Figs. 14.21–14.23**).

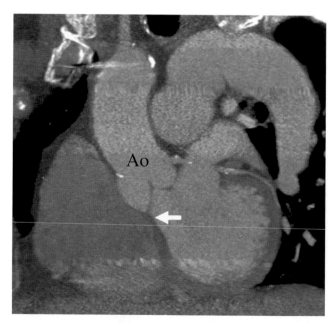

Figure 14.21 *An oblique coronal views demonstrates an intact ventricular septum after patch repair (arrow) and the appearance that the aorta (Ao) that "overrides" the septum in this congenital heart defect.*

(A)

(B)

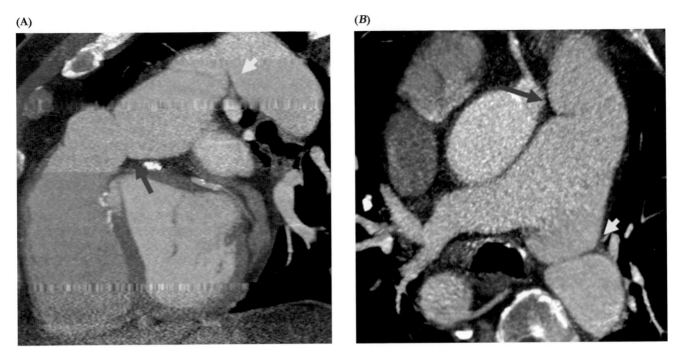

Figure 14.22   *Oblique sagittal (**A**) and axial (**B**) views demonstrate multiple levels of distal obstruction that may contribute to worsening systolic function of the right ventricle. There is an area of stenosis in the proximal main pulmonary artery* (red arrows). *In addition, a thorough assessment of the distal pulmonary artery architecture is important in patients with prior palliative Blalock–Taussig shunts. These shunts often lead to distortion of the pulmonary artery architecture. In this case, there is a stenosis of the proximal left pulmonary artery* (yellow arrows) *at the prior site of shunt placement.*

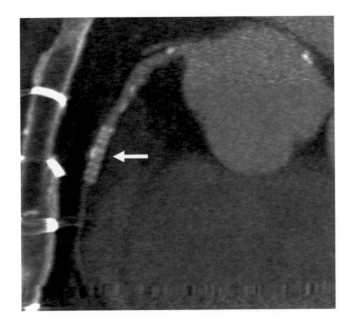

Figure 14.23   *Oblique sagittal view demonstrates patency of the right coronary artery (RCA) stent* (arrow) *with areas of plaque in the proximal RCA.*

TETRALOGY OF FALLOT AND PULMONARY
ATRESIA

Clinical Case 12

A 26-year-old male with tetralogy of Fallot and
pulmonary atresia underwent a valved RV–PA
conduit. He had been lost to follow-up and now
presented to the Adolescent and Adult Congenital
Heart Disease Clinic with worsening shortness of
breath and atrial fibrillation. In addition to a
cardiac MRI, a complimentary CT examination
was also performed to evaluate the distal PA
architecture and coronary artery anatomy
(**Figs. 14.24–14.27**).

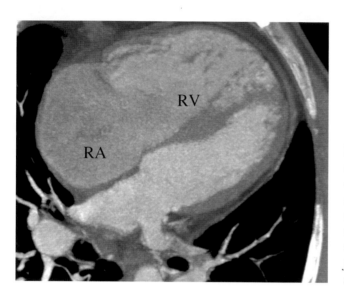

Figure 14.24 *Oblique short axis view demonstrates the
severely dilated right atrium (RA) and ventricle (RV) in
comparison to the relatively normal appearance of the
left-sided structures. The RV ejection fraction by CT measured 23%. A thorough assessment of functional abnormalities contributing to RV enlargement and concomitant dysfunction is warranted as correction of underlying
functional abnormalities may preserve or improve RV
systolic dysfunction.*

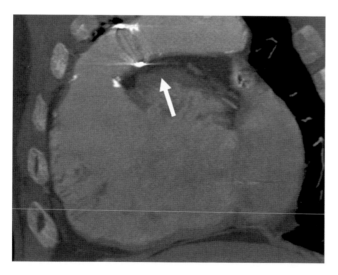

Figure 14.25 *An oblique sagittal view demonstrates no
evidence of residual valvular* (white arrow), *subvalvular,
or infundibular hypertrophy that could account for the
changes in right ventricle size or function.*

(B)

(A)

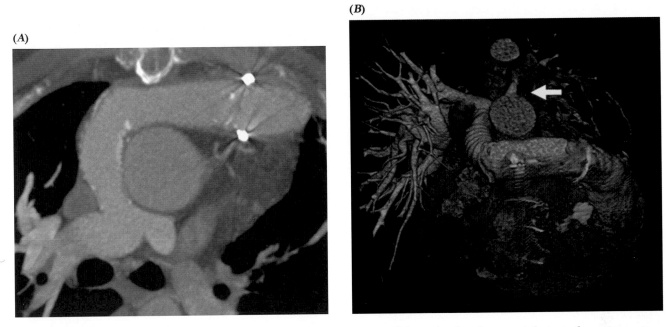

Figure 14.26 *An oblique axial view demonstrates the patency of the valved right ventricle-to-pulmonary artery conduit* (**A**). *A volume-rendered reconstruction* (**B**) *suggests a stenosis of the left pulmonary artery* (arrow). *In addition, there is a paucity of distal pulmonary artery vessels in contrast to the normal appearance of the distal right pulmonary artery branches.*

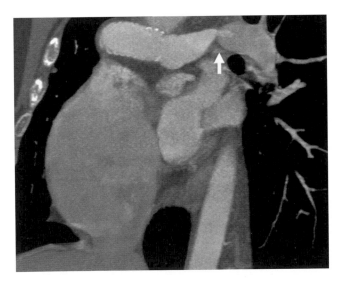

Figure 14.27 *This oblique sagittal view identifies a critical area of left pulmonary artery stenosis* (arrow) *that may contribute to the severe right ventricular enlargement and consequent systolic dysfunction in this patient.*

TRANSPOSITION OF THE GREAT VESSELS

Clinical Case 13

A 24-year-old male with a history of d-transposition of the great arteries who underwent Mustard repair (atrial switch procedure), and sick sinus syndrome requiring a dual chamber pacemaker presented for a routine follow-up evaluation. The dual chamber pacemaker precludes assessment of anatomy and function with cardiac MRI and therefore this patient underwent a cardiac CT to evaluate patency of the pulmonary venous and systemic venous atria as well as for the functional assessment of the pulmonary (morphologic LV) and systemic (morphologic RV) ventricles (**Figs. 14.28–14.31**).

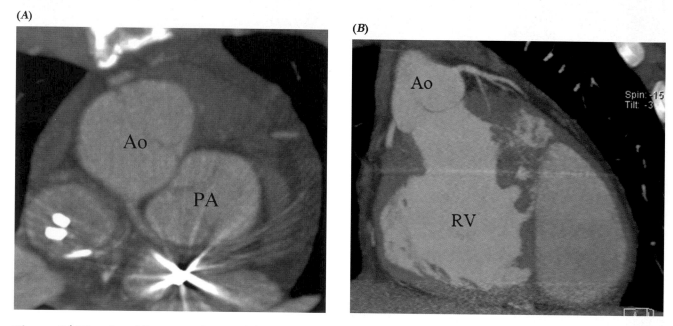

Figure 14.28 *An oblique axial view (**A**) shows the typical configuration of the great vessels in patients with d-transposition of the great arteries with the aorta (Ao) anterior and rightward of the pulmonary artery (PA). Determination of great vessels is simplified by identification of the ostia of the coronary arteries, thus identifying the aorta. This embryologic abnormality results in ventriculo-arterial discordance, with the aorta arising from the right ventricle (RV) and the pulmonary artery arising from the left ventricle (**B**).*

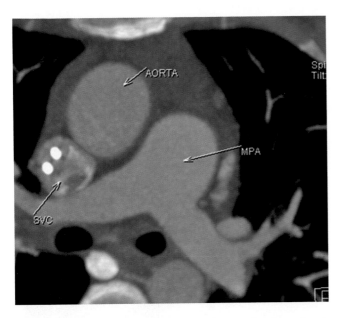

Figure 14.29 *This oblique axial view further classifies the relationship of the great vessels as the posterior and leftward structure bifurcates to the right and left pulmonary arteries successfully identifying this vessel correctly as the pulmonary artery. The atrial and ventricular wires are easily identified in the superior vena cava (SVC). Abbreviation: MPA, main pulmonary artery.*

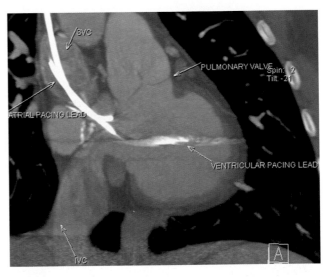

Figure 14.30 *The Mustard repair, or atrial switch procedure, directs the superior vena cava (SVC) and inferior vena cava (IVC) to the pulmonary or morphologic left ventricle. Again, ventriculo-arterial discordance is present as the pulmonary valve is in continuity with the left ventricle. This view is helpful to identify obstruction at the superior or inferior aspect of the systemic venous baffle.*

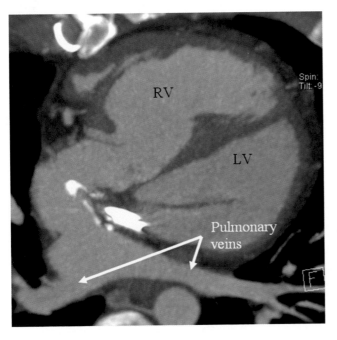

Figure 14.31 *The Mustard repair also redirects pulmonary venous flow to the systemic or morphologic right ventricle (RV). CT is particularly helpful in identifying any obstruction to pulmonary venous inflow. The left and right lower pulmonary veins (arrows) seen in this oblique axial view are directed through an unobstructed baffle to the trabeculated right ventricle.*

DOUBLE-OUTLET RV

Clinical Case 14

A 28-year-old female with double-outlet RV (DORV) underwent repair with a RV–PA conduit and presented for routine follow-up evaluation. Cardiac MRI identified severe conduit stenosis. Cardiac CT was obtained to assess calcification of the conduit and evaluate the distal pulmonary arteries prior to transcatheter intervention (**Figs. 14.32–14.34**).

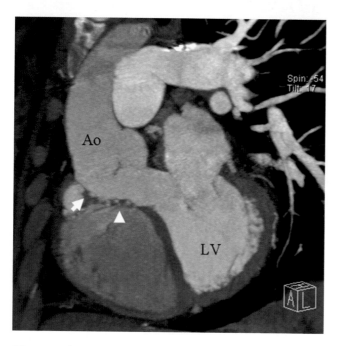

Figure 14.32 *An oblique sagittal view demonstrates the rightward displacement of the aorta (Ao). In certain types of double-outlet right ventricle a biventricular repair can be performed. The patch utilized to close the ventricular septal defect* (arrows) *routes flow from the left ventricle (LV) to the aorta.*

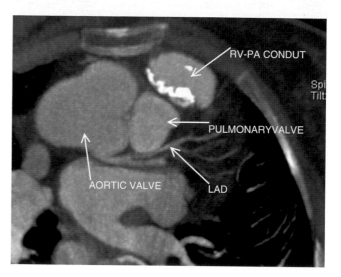

Figure 14.33 *This oblique axial demonstrates the side-by-side position of the great arteries with the aorta rightward (identified by the left anterior descending coronary artery arising from this great vessel) of the hypoplastic appearing pulmonary valve. The right ventricle-to-pulmonary artery (RV-PA) conduit demonstrates focal, moderate calcification. Abbreviation: LAD, left anterior descending coronary artery.*

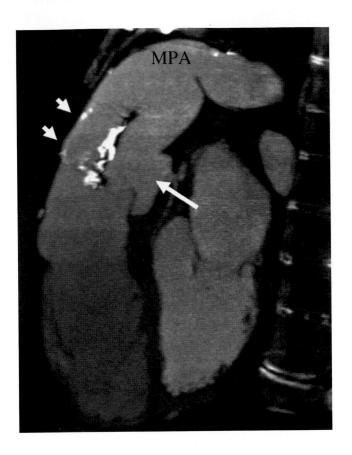

MPA

Figure 14.34 *An oblique sagittal view demonstrates the native right ventricular outflow tract* (arrow) *and the calcified appearance of the right ventricle-to-pulmonary artery (RV–PA) conduit* (arrowheads). *In addition there is a fold in the distal main pulmonary artery (MPA) after the anastomosis of the conduit and the native right ventricular outflow tract.*

CLINICAL CASE 15

A 23-year-old female with DORV initially underwent a left-sided Blalock–Taussig shunt followed by complete repair. Later, she was found to have left PA stenosis requiring implantation of a Genesis stent and coil occlusion of the Blalock–Taussig shunt. She presented for a prepregnancy screening evaluation in the Adolescent and Young Adult Congenital Heart Disease Clinic. Artifact created by the coils utilized to occlude the Blalock–Taussig shunt prevented a thorough assessment of her intracardiac anatomy with cardiac MRI and therefore she underwent a complementary cardiac CT to assess her intracardiac anatomy, pulmonary anatomy, stent patency, and left and right ventricular function (**Figs. 14.35–14.38**).

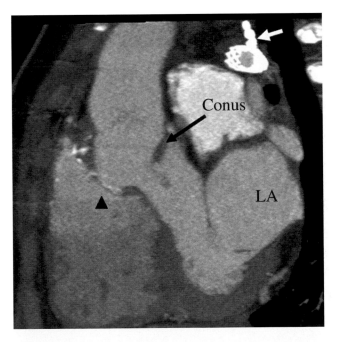

Conus

LA

Figure 14.35 *An oblique sagittal view demonstrates the complex intracardiac anatomy after surgical repair. Failure of leftward shift and differential absorption of the primitive conus* (black arrow) *results in persistance of both great arteries from the right ventricle. Despite surgical repair with patch closure of the ventricular septal defect* (arrowhead), *this conus may create subaortic obstruction and ensuing pressure gradient. In addition, the coils used to occlude the shunt are also seen* (white arrow).

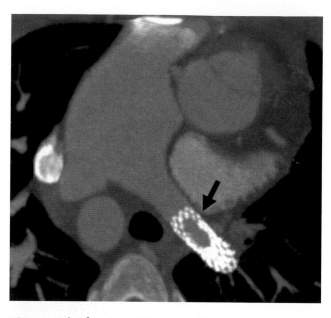

Figure 14.36 *An oblique axial view demonstrates the dilated main pulmonary artery with a maximal diameter of 44 mm and the stent in the proximal left pulmonary artery (arrow).*

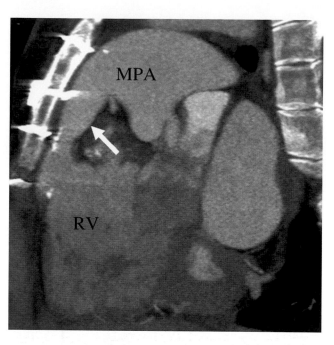

Figure 14.37 *The narrowed right ventricle-to-pulmonary artery (RV–PA) conduit may explain the dilated appearance of the main pulmonary artery (MPA).*

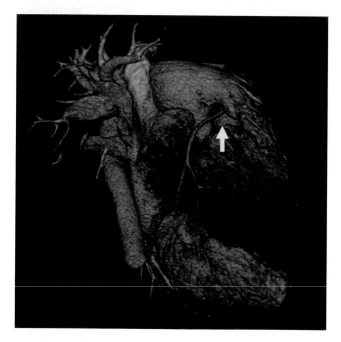

Figure 14.38 *A volume rendered three-dimensional reconstruction importantly identifies the right coronary artery traversing between the native right ventricular outflow tract and the right ventricle-to-pulmonary artery (RV–PA) conduit, which has significant implications if this young woman were to undergo surgical revision of the RV–PA conduit in the future.*

MISCELLANEOUS

COR TRIATRIATUM

Clinical Case 16

A 40-year-old male with a history of an ostium primum ASD and cleft mitral valve previously underwent patch closure of the ASD and mitral valve cleft repair, hypertension, and tobacco addiction presented with shortness of breath. A cardiac CT was performed as part of the evaluation of dyspnea to evaluate the underlying anatomy and assess coronary artery atherosclerosis (**Fig. 14.39**).

(A)

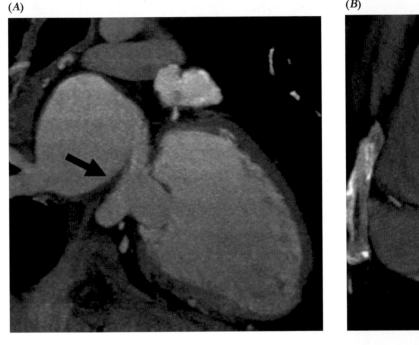

(B)

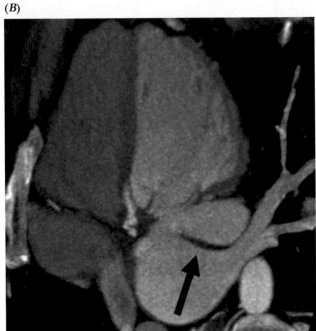

(C)

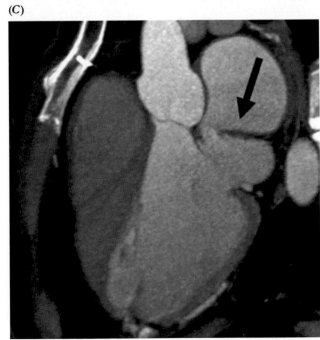

Figure 14.39 *A two-chamber (**A**), four-chamber (**B**), and three-chamber view (**C**) all demonstrate a discrete ridge of tissue (arrows) above the plane of the mitral valve consistent with cor triatriatum sinister, accounting for the shortness of breath in this patient despite prior surgical repair.*

CORONARY-CAMERAL FISTULAE

Clinical Case 17

A 14-year-old female with a history of multiple coronary-cameral fistulae presented for a routine follow-up evaluation. A cardiac CT was performed to assess the coronary arteries (**Fig. 14.40**).

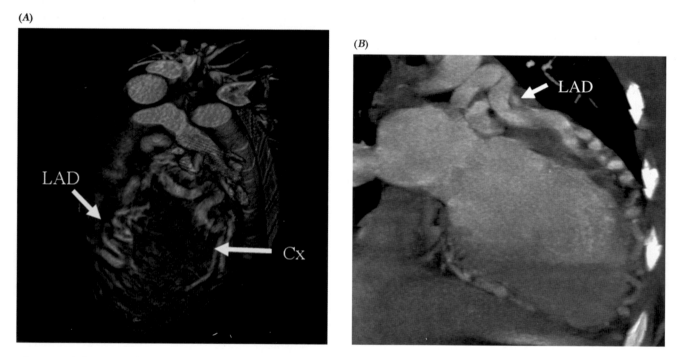

Figure 14.40 *A volume rendered three-dimensional reconstruction (**A**) and oblique sagittal view (**B**) demonstrate the diffusely aneurismal appearance of the left anterior descending (LAD) measuring 11mm in diameter and circumflex (Cx) artery measuring 10mm in diameter proximally.*

CLINICAL PEARLS

- The number of adults with congenital heart disease continues to increase. Many of these patients may require surgical or transcatheter interventions as a result of their prior palliative repairs. Complex anatomy commonly seen in this patient population places rigorous demands on current noninvasive tools available to completely and accurately assess this population.

- Traditional imaging modalities are limited in this patient population as a result of chest wall deformities and obesity. CTA provides a novel method to assess these patients who may have contraindications to CMR examinations and metallic implants that create signal void with CMR imaging. The speed of acquisition is helpful in patients with decompensated heart failure and cyanosis.

- CTA provides insight into the structural cardiovascular changes in adults with congenital heart disease caused by underlying morphologic abnormalities.

- Left and right ventricular volumes, ejection fraction, and cavity dimensions can be quantified with CTA, and results are comparable to those obtained with other cardiac imaging modalities.

- CTA overcomes the limitations of angiography in this patient population as it provides a detailed 3D assesssment of the coronary artery anatomy, which is often anomalous in this population, in relation to the great arteries and other surrounding structures.

- CTA is frequently utilized in the pre- and post-interventional setting. Ultimately, this reduces the amount of contrast and radiation exposure at the time of intervention and provides a means to assess transcatheter results.

- Innovations and advances in CTA imaging to detect earlier abnormalities requiring transcatheter and/or surgical interventions may lead to improved outcomes in this complex patient population.

Index